10-MINUTE

FITNESS

TRANSFORM YOUR DAY WITH QUICK WORKOUTS

BY

PAUL CANNON

DISCLAIMER

This book is intended for educational purposes only. The information provided within is designed to offer guidance and inspiration for incorporating 10-minute workouts into your daily routine to support your overall well-being.

Please be aware that individual results may vary, and the effectiveness of any fitness program depends on various factors, including your current fitness level, health status, and adherence to the program. Before starting any new exercise regimen, it is advisable to consult with a qualified healthcare professional, particularly if you have underlying health concerns or medical conditions.

The author and publisher of this book do not assume any liability for injuries, losses, or damages that may occur as a result of implementing the exercises or advice provided in this book. It is essential to exercise caution, listen to your body, and seek professional guidance if needed.

Remember that the path to fitness and health is a personal journey, and it's important to prioritize safety and individual well-being above all else.

TABLE OF CONTENTS

INTRODUCTION 8

CHAPTER 1 11

THE TIME-CRUNCHED LIFE & PHILOSOPHY 11

10-Minute Workout Concept.............................14

Science of Short Workouts...............................15

Benefits of HIIT and Tabata............................17

Debunking Exercise Myths 19

Real-Life Integration 21

Summary 25

CHAPTER 2 27

SETTING REALISTIC FITNESS GOALS 27

The importance of setting achievable fitness goals...29

How to apply the SMART criteria to fitness............31

Stress the importance of consistency over intensity for long-term success 34

Summary 36

CHAPTER 3 ....**38**

CREATING YOUR 10 -MINUTE WORKOUT PLAN...38

Strategies for integrating workouts into daily routines 40

Tips on staying committed to a 10-minute daily exercise plan 42

Ways to adapt workout times and types to match energy and schedules 45

Summary 48

CHAPTER 4 ....**50**

WORKOUT 1 - FULL-BODY BLAST **50**

Detailed plan for a 10-minute full-body workout 51

The muscles worked and the benefits of each movement 57

Summary 61

CHAPTER 5 ....**63**

WORKOUT 2 - CHEST AND ARMS SCULPT **63**

Focused 10-minute routine for the chest and biceps .64

Tips and dumbbell technique guidance 67

How to modify exercises for different fitness levels .69

Summary 72

CHAPTER 6 ....**74**

WORKOUT 3 - CORE STRENGTHENING CIRCUIT .74

A quick, intense core workout routine 75

Include instructions for exercises that target the entire core 78

The importance of core strength for overall fitness ..80

Summary 83

CHAPTER 7 ....**85**

WORKOUT 4 - POWER LEGS **85**

A 10-minute workout focused on leg strength and endurance..86

Exercise variations for different intensity levels 89

The importance of leg workouts for metabolic health 92

Summary 94

CHAPTER 8 ....**97**

WORKOUT 5 - TOTAL BALANCE **97**

Combine previous exercises into a balanced routine 98

Focus on exercises that promote stability and muscle coordination...101

Summary 107

CHAPTER 9 ....**109**

FROM MINUTES TO MOMENTUM....................**109**

Short workouts into a consistent routine 110

How to increase workout duration progressively?..113

The psychological benefits of regular, achievable workouts 115

Summary 118

CHAPTER 10 ....**120**

MANAGING MUSCLE FATIGUE AND RECOVERY **120**

The importance of rest and recovery in a workout regimen..121

Tips for recognizing and managing muscle fatigue 123

Strategies for active recovery on rest days..............126

Summary 129

CHAPTER 11 ....**131**

THE BENEFITS OF CONSISTENCY **131**

The long-term health benefits of regular exercise...134

How consistency in workouts can lead to improved physical and mental health 136

How small daily efforts accumulate over time........139

Summary 142

CHAPTER 12 ....**144**

NUTRITION AND THE 10 - MINUTE WORKOUT **144**

The role of hydration, protein intake, and quick energy sources 147

Summary 152

CHAPTER 13 ....**154**

YOUR NEXT STEPS..**154**

Tips for maintaining motivation and measuring progress 156

How to advance to new fitness challenges over time? 160

INTRODUCTION

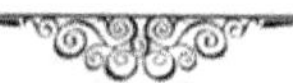

Imagine you're at the end of another day, and despite your best intentions, there wasn't a spare moment for that trip to the gym. With meetings that ran long, a lunch hour filled with errands, and a to-do list that never seems to get any shorter, where's the space for fitness? I've been there, too. As someone who's juggled multiple roles and responsibilities, I understand the challenge of fitting in a workout. That's why I wrote "10-Minute Fitness."

This book answers the common belief that there's not enough time for exercise. I'll tell you a secret: effective workouts don't have to consume hours of your day. Ten minutes, the time it might take you to scroll through your news feed or wait in line for your morning espresso, is enough to start a transformation.

Over the years, I've watched friends, even I struggle with the idea of fitness being synonymous with long gym sessions. That misconception is about to change. With "10-Minute Fitness," you're holding a guide that demystifies the art of the quick workout, designed for the ultra-busy, the tired, and everyone in between.

Why 10 minutes, you ask? It's achievable, sustainable, and, most importantly, scientifically proven to be effective. You'll learn that short bursts of activity can improve your heart health, boost your metabolism, and build strength just as well as those extended sessions, if not better. We'll break down the latest research into bite-sized, actionable advice you can use from day one.

We'll also tackle goal setting, not the New Year's resolution kind that fades by February, but real, life-compatible goals. We're talking about the small, daily victories that add to massive changes over time. Whether improving your endurance, shedding a few pounds, or simply feeling more energized, "10-Minute Fitness" shows you how to get there, one step at a time.

In these pages, I'll share five different 10-minute workouts that you can do anywhere - no fancy gym equipment needed. We'll cover all bases, from your legs to your core, right up to your arms and chest. Each exercise is designed to maximize your time, so every minute counts.

The benefits they extend far beyond what you might expect. Sure, you'll see physical changes, but the boost to your mood, the clarity of your mind, and the extra spring in your step will convince you of the power of short workouts. I've seen people transform their days and, ultimately, their lives with just these quick sessions.

Finally, we'll look at how to keep the momentum going. I'm talking about turning these quick workouts into a consistent habit that leads to longer, more challenging sessions as your fitness improves. It's all about building up at your own pace, with "10-Minute Fitness" as your companion.

In short, if you've ever felt too busy to be healthy, this book is for you. So, let's lace up those sneakers and turn your can't s into cans and your dreams into plans. It's time to fit fitness into your life, 10 minutes at a time.

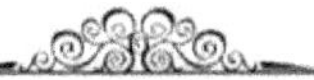

CHAPTER 1

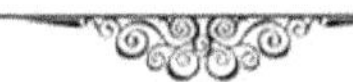

THE TIME-CRUNCHED LIFE & PHILOSOPHY

Lost time is never found again

- Benjamin Franklin

In today's world, where our schedules are jam-packed from dawn to dusk, squeezing in time for exercise often feels like an unsolvable riddle. We're all caught in the whirlwind of daily responsibilities—rushing to meet work deadlines, managing household chores, and fulfilling family obligations. Amidst this chaos, dedicating a significant chunk of time to workout sessions seems like a luxury few can afford.

This predicament has become a universal theme in our modern lifestyles. It's not just about the struggle to stay fit; it's about the constant battle against time. The irony is stark: exercise is crucial for our health and well-being, yet we find ourselves trapped in a cycle where time for physical activity is perpetually pushed to the bottom of our to-do lists. The result is a nagging sense of guilt and the unwelcome consequences of a sedentary lifestyle.

The conventional view of exercise often adds to this challenge. There's a widespread belief that effective workouts demand long hours at the gym, sweating on treadmills, or lifting weights. This notion, deeply ingrained in our collective psyche, makes it harder to see exercise as something achievable within the constraints of our busy lives.

However, what if we could shift this perspective? What if exercise didn't have to be a time-consuming affair but could be a series of quick, intense bursts of activity seamlessly woven into our day? This idea is based on wishful thinking and a practical approach backed by science and real-life success stories. It's about recognizing that a few minutes of focused physical activity can be as beneficial as prolonged workout sessions.

This understanding brings us to short, efficient workouts—a solution tailored to our time-starved existence. Imagine replacing the hour-long gym session, which seems impossible to fit into your day, with a 10-minute high-intensity workout that you can do in your living room, office, or even in a park. These mini-workouts are a compromise and an intelligent strategy to maintain fitness without disrupting our hectic schedules.

The beauty of these short workouts lies in their simplicity and flexibility. You don't need expensive gym memberships or fancy equipment. A small space, a few minutes, and the willingness to push you are all it takes. Whether it's a quick cardio session before breakfast, a brisk strength-training routine during your lunch break, or stretches before bed, these snippets of exercise can add significant health benefits.

Incorporating these brief but effective workouts into our daily routine is a realistic and sustainable approach to fitness. It's about maximizing our limited time and recognizing that every minute counts. As we navigate the chapters ahead, we'll explore how to make this concept a practical reality, offering guidance and inspiration to transform how we think about exercise and time management. The goal is simple yet profound: to foster a healthier lifestyle that respects the constraints of our busy lives.

10-Minute Workout Concept

Fitting exercise into a busy schedule can seem impossible. But what if we could break that barrier with something as simple as 10-minute workouts? These aren't just quick fixes; they're a complete rethinking of how we view exercise. Instead of seeing it as something that needs hours at the gym, we start to see it as short bursts of activity that can easily fit into our day.

The idea is straightforward. You take a small window of time, right before you shower in the morning or during that mid-afternoon slump when you'd usually grab a coffee, and turn it into your mini-workout zone. In just 10 minutes, you can do high-energy exercises like jumping jacks, push-ups, or quick sprints. The key is to keep the intensity high; every second counts since the time is short.

This approach is more than just a time-saver. It's about making exercise feel less daunting and more doable. When you think about sweating it out for an hour, saying, "I'll do it tomorrow is easy." But 10 minutes?

That's about the time you'd spend scrolling through your phone or waiting for your pasta to cook. It's a small enough commitment that doesn't feel overwhelming, yet long enough to get your heart rate up and give you a good workout.

And the benefits are surprising. These short workouts can boost your mood, give you energy, and improve your focus for the rest of the day. They're also great for your health. Short workouts can improve heart health; help with weight management, and even build muscle strength.

The best part is you don't need any special equipment or a gym membership. If you're traveling, you can do these exercises in your living room, office, or even a hotel room. It's all about using what you have and making the most of your time.

So, the next time you feel like you can't fit exercise into your day, remember the 10-minute workout. It's a small step, but it can significantly change how you think and manage your health and fitness in a busy world.

Science of Short Workouts

The science behind short workouts, especially high-intensity interval training or HIIT, is fascinating and a game-changer for many. HIIT focuses on quick bursts of intense activity and subsequent brief rest periods. It's like sprinting as fast as you can for a minute, walking a bit, and repeating the cycle. This type of workout can be done in about 15 to 30 minutes, but it packs a punch in terms of effectiveness.

One of the most incredible things about HIIT is its continuing to burn calories long after you're done working out. This happens because intense exercise pushes your body's repair cycles into hyperdrive. So, even when you're done with your workout and sitting on your couch, your body still works hard, burns calories, and builds muscle.

Another great thing about HIIT is that it's flexible. You can do it with many different exercises, like running, biking, jumping rope, or even bodyweight exercises like push-ups and squats. This means you can quickly adapt it to your fitness level and available space or equipment.

What's more, research shows that HIIT can significantly improve cardiovascular health. It's like giving your heart a good workout, making it more robust and efficient at pumping blood. It's also great for improving endurance and reducing blood sugar levels.

But the best part? HIIT is super time-efficient. When it might take you to drive to the gym, you can complete a full HIIT workout right at home. This makes it a perfect fit for anyone needing help carving out time for longer exercise sessions.

So, when you think about HIIT, imagine giving your body and health a significant boost in just a tiny slice of your day. It's a powerful way to exercise and fits right into our busy lives, showing us that you don't need to spend hours in the gym to get fit and healthy.

Tabata

Tabata is a form of high-intensity interval training (HIIT) that has gained widespread popularity due to its efficiency and effectiveness. Dr. Izumi Tabata, a Japanese scientist and researcher from the National Institute of Fitness and Sports in Tokyo, created it in the late 1990s.

Benefits of HIIT and Tabata

HIIT and Tabata workouts might sound like another fitness trend, but they're packed with profound health benefits. These workouts are about getting maximum results in minimal time, making them a perfect fit for anyone with a busy schedule.

So, what's so great about these workouts? HIIT, which stands for High-Intensity Interval Training, is a super-efficient way to boost your heart health. It makes your heart pump hard for short bursts, which improves cardiovascular fitness. Plus, it's a real calorie burner. Because of the high intensity, you burn many calories quickly, and your body continues to burn calories even after you finish working out.

Then there's Tabata, a form of HIIT that's even more condensed. It's a four-minute workout where you go all out for 20 seconds, rest for 10 seconds, and then repeat. Although it might seem too good to be true, science supports this. Tabata is not only great for burning calories but also for boosting your metabolism. This means you'll burn more calories when you're not working out.

Another big plus of these workouts is their flexibility. You can do a HIIT or Tabata workout with just about any exercise—running, cycling, bodyweight exercises, you name it. This means you can easily tailor them to your fitness level and the space or equipment you have.

The best part about HIIT and Tabata is how they fit into a busy life. You don't need to dedicate an hour or more to get a good workout. With these methods, you can get solid, practical training in just a few minutes. This makes sticking to a regular exercise routine much more accessible, even when life gets hectic.

In short, HIIT and Tabata offer a way to get fit, improve heart health, and burn calories efficiently, all in a time frame that suits even the busiest schedules. They're a practical, effective approach to fitness that can make a real difference in your health and well-being.

Debunking Exercise Myths

There's a big myth about exercise: that you need to spend hours in the gym or on a long run to get fit. But that's not true, and understanding this can be a game-changer for many of us. You can dedicate less than half your day to working out to see results.

This myth has made many people feel like they can't fit exercise into their lives. If you think you need a spare two hours to get a good workout, it's easy to give up and not exercise. But here's the good news: shorter workouts can be just as effective—sometimes even more so—as longer ones.

It's all about how you use the time. High-intensity workouts, like HIIT, make every minute count. Instead of a leisurely hour-long jog, you could do a 20-minute HIIT session and get more benefits: better cardiovascular fitness, more calories burned, and a more significant boost to your metabolism.

This new understanding flips the old idea of what a workout looks like. It means that you can still find time to exercise even on your busiest days. Do you have 10 minutes before you shower and head out for the day? That's enough for a quick HIIT session. Are you waiting for dinner to cook? Perfect time for a short bodyweight workout.

Letting go of the myth that longer is always better can make exercise more accessible and doable for everyone. It's a shift in mindset that opens up a whole new world of possibilities for staying fit and healthy, even amid our busy, often chaotic lives.

Real-Life Integration

Getting short workouts into your daily life might seem tricky, but it's all about finding those little pockets of time and making them count. First off, look at your typical day. Where are those moments you might be waiting around or doing something passive, like watching TV? Those are the perfect times to squeeze in a quick workout.

Start with your morning routine. At the same time, waiting for your coffee to brew or right after waking up, you can fit in simple exercises like squats, push-ups, or jumping jacks. It's a great way to energize your body for the day ahead.

Then there's the lunch break. Most of us get some time here, often used for scrolling through our phones. How about swapping a few minutes of screen time for a brisk walk or a quick set of stair climbing? It's good for your body and can also clear your mind and boost your mood.

Evenings can be another great opportunity. During dinner's cooking, or in those minutes you'd usually spend settling down on the sofa, why not throw in a short burst of high-intensity activity? You could do a quick circuit of bodyweight exercises, or if you have a jump rope, that's a great way to get your heart pumping fast.

It's also about making it a habit. Try setting a reminder on your phone or sticking a Post-it note somewhere visible. These little cues can help turn these short exercise sessions into a regular part of your routine.

Remember, the goal isn't to exhaust you but to be consistent. Its okay if you only manage a few minutes some days; it's still better than nothing and keeps the habit going. Over time, these tiny bits of activity can make a big difference in how you feel and your overall fitness.

The key is to keep it simple and doable. You don't need to gear up for a marathon; get moving in whatever way fits into your life. Before you know it, these short workouts will become a natural part of your day, and you'll wonder how you ever did without them.

When it comes to health and fitness, every minute does count. There's no point in trying if you don't have a whole hour to dedicate to a workout. But this mindset overlooks the actual value of time, especially in our fast-paced world, where every second is precious.

The truth is that even the briefest moments dedicated to physical activity can significantly impact our health. Think about the small choices you make daily - taking the stairs instead of the elevator, taking a quick walk during your lunch break, or even standing more often. These choices add up, contributing to a healthier lifestyle without demanding vast chunks of time from your busy schedule.

Short workouts offer a practical solution, like a quick 10-minute HIIT session. They allow us to make the most of our limited time, showing that you don't need to block out hours of your day to stay fit. This approach to exercise is about being innovative and efficient - getting the most health benefits in the shortest amount of time.

The beauty of these mini-workouts is that they can fit into the nooks and crannies of your day. They don't require a massive shift in your daily routine or lifestyle. Instead, they seamlessly integrate into the schedule you already have. For example, a few minutes of high-intensity exercise in the morning can wake you up better than a cup of coffee. A brisk walk or stretching during a break at work can re-energize you for the rest of your day.

Adopting this mindset also helps us overcome the all-or-nothing approach to fitness. Instead of feeling guilty for not spending an hour in the gym, we can feel good about the small but powerful efforts we make each day. It's about celebrating the little victories and recognizing they are steps toward better health.

Moreover, this approach can be a great motivator. It builds momentum when you start seeing and feeling the benefits of these short workouts. You begin to realize that staying active is more manageable than it seemed and that you have the time to care for your body. This realization can be incredibly empowering.

Incorporating exercise into your daily life doesn't have to be a grand gesture. It's about maximizing your time, no matter how limited. It's about changing our perception of a workout and understanding that every minute dedicated to our health is valuable.

As we wrap up, it's important to remember that fitness is a personal journey. What works for one person might not work for another. The key is to find what fits into your life and makes you feel good. Whether it's a few minutes of yoga in the morning, a quick jog in the evening, or several short bouts of activity scattered throughout your day, what matters is that you're moving and taking care of your health.

So, let's embrace the idea that in health and fitness, every minute counts. It's not about having more time; it's about maximizing our time. With this approach, we can all find ways to stay active, healthy, and fit, no matter how busy our lives are.

Summary

- Emphasizes the importance of valuing each minute regarding fitness and health, challenging the notion that only long workout sessions are practical.
- Highlights how minor daily activities, like taking stairs, short walks, or standing tasks, can contribute significantly to a healthier lifestyle.

- Discusses the benefits of 10-minute high-intensity workouts and their ability to fit into busy schedules without requiring large time blocks.

- It focuses on the efficiency of short, intense workouts, offering maximum health benefits in minimal time.

- It shows how easy it is to incorporate mini workouts into the day without overhauling one's schedule, such as quick exercises in the morning or during work breaks.

- Addresses the needs to move away from the perception that only long workouts are worthwhile, recognizing the value of shorter, more consistent efforts.

- Explains how starting with small, manageable workouts can build motivation and create a positive feedback loop.

- It reminds us that fitness is a personal journey and what works for one may not work for another; the key is to find activities that fit individual lifestyles and preferences.

- Encourages the adoption of a mindset that seeks to make the most of available time, demonstrating that staying active and healthy is possible, even with a busy schedule.

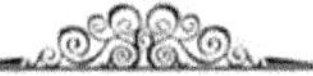

CHAPTER 2

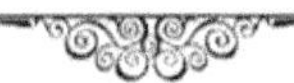

SETTING REALISTIC FITNESS GOALS

A goal properly set is halfway reached.

– Zig Ziglar

Embarking on a fitness journey without a destination is like setting sail without a compass. It's essential to know where you're going and make sure it's a place you can realistically reach. Setting fitness goals isn't about dreaming big and then stumbling on reality; it's about carving a doable path that will keep you motivated daily.

Let's get down to brass tacks when juggling work, family, and countless other responsibilities; your fitness goals must fit into your life, not the other way around. This means setting targets that respect your time constraints and energy levels. It's not about training for a marathon when you can barely squeeze in a daily walk. It's about finding that sweet spot where your aspirations meet your schedule.

This chapter will guide you to setting goals as realistic as they are rewarding. Think of it as your blueprint for success. We will look at what it means to set SMART goals – Specific, Measurable, Achievable, Relevant, and Time-bound. This isn't just a fancy acronym; it's a proven strategy that transforms vague wishes into tangible targets.

Setting realistic fitness goals also means knowing yourself. It's about being honest about what you're willing to commit to and what just wishful thinking is. There's no room for self-deception here, only self-awareness. Because when you set goals that genuinely resonate with you, you're more likely to stick with them.

And remember, setting goals is not a one-and-done deal. It's an ongoing process. Life changes and your goals should be flexible enough to accommodate those changes. The key is to keep them challenging yet achievable. That way, every little victory keeps you moving forward, and every setback is just a slight detour, not the end of the road.

In this chapter, we'll journey through the goal-setting process, ensuring that by the end, you'll know where you want to go with your fitness and have a clear and achievable map to get there.

The importance of setting achievable fitness goals

Setting achievable fitness goals is like quietly plotting a revolution against the "I'll do it tomorrow" mindset that keeps us stuck in a rut. It's a commitment to progress, not perfection. When we set goals within our reach, we're not just dreaming about a fitter self but planning a route to get there.

Think about it this way: if you want to climb a mountain, you wouldn't just stare at the peak and hope for the best. You'd start with the foothills, get used to the climb, and work your way up. The same goes for fitness. If you've barely laced up a pair of sneakers in the last year, aiming to run a marathon next month sets you up for disappointment. But a goal to take a brisk 10-minute walks every day? Now, that's something you can immediately grab hold of. Why are achievable goals so important? For starters, they're good for your confidence. Every time you meet a small goal, it's a win, and that success fuels your desire to tackle the next one. It's like a chain reaction of motivation. If you manage to do those 10-minute walks, maybe next you'll try 15. Before you know it, you could be jogging those same minutes. The progression is natural, encouraging, and—most importantly—doable.

Another crucial reason is the risk of burnout. When you set a mammoth goal, the energy and time it demands can quickly become overwhelming. And when we're overwhelmed, we tend to give up. Small, achievable goals are kinder to your daily energy reserves. You can fit them in, do them well, and still have juice left for the rest of your day. Achievable goals are also easier to measure, and that's important because what gets measured gets done. It's satisfying to tick off a plan that's clear and defined. Did you do your 10-minute walk today? Check. That's measurable. "Get fit" is an amorphous aim that's hard to pin down and even harder to celebrate.

Let's remember life's curveballs. Setting realistic goals means adapting to the unexpected without losing sight of your fitness aims. Got an extra-busy week at work? A 10-minute workout can slide right in. There's no need to forego fitness because you think it's all or nothing. Lastly, achieving smaller goals is plain good for your health. You're not pushing your body to the brink. Instead, you're building a habit, the cornerstone of lasting health. With each small goal, you're paving the way to a lifestyle that naturally embraces movement. In essence, achievable fitness goals are your milestones on the road to a healthier life. They're about making promises to yourself that you can keep, taking the stairs instead of the elevator and acknowledging that while the destination matters, the journey – one step at a time – is equally important.

How to apply the SMART criteria to fitness

The SMART criteria are like a secret recipe for creating goals that aren't just daydreams but plans with a punch. It's about giving your fitness aspirations a backbone, strengthening them to withstand the daily grind. So, let's break down this recipe and see how each ingredient contributes to cooking up successful fitness goals.

First up is 'Specific.' To make your goals specific, you've got to be clear about what you want. Let's say you want to improve your fitness. That's a good start, but it's as vague as saying you want to travel. Where to? How? Instead, pinpoint exactly what you're after. You may want to be able to run 5 kilometers or fit into those Jenes that have been quietly judging you from the back of your closet. That's specific.

Next, we've got 'Measurable.' You need to know when you've hit your target. If your goal is as specific as running 5 kilometers, you'll know you've achieved it when you can hit that distance without feeling like you need a new set of lungs. Making your goal measurable means you can track your progress, which significantly boosts your motivation.

Then there's 'Achievable'. This is where you need a good dose of reality. If you've been a couch fan for years, deciding to hit the gym every day at dawn suddenly might be biting off more than you can chew. Achievable means setting goals that stretch you but are still within the realm of possibility. Think about what you can realistically commit to and make that your target.

'Relevant' is your next ingredient. This is all about ensuring your goal matters to you because you won't stick to it if it doesn't. If you're not a morning person, don't kid yourself into thinking you'll suddenly become one for the sake of exercise. Choose a fitness goal that fits your lifestyle, values, and what you enjoy.

Lastly, we have 'Time-bound.' Deadlines aren't just for work projects; they work wonders for fitness goals. They give you a timeframe to focus on, which helps keep procrastination at bay. Whether it's a month or six, set a deadline for your goal to keep the fire under your feet.

Now, how do you put all these ingredients together? Let's say you want to start running. A SMART goal would be: "I want to run a total of 5 kilometers in one go, without stopping, within the next three months." It's specific (run 5 kilometers), measurable (in one go, without stopping), achievable (you've given yourself time to train up to it), relevant (you've chosen running because you love the outdoors), and time-bound (three months from now).

That's the essence of applying the SMART criteria to fitness. It's about getting granular with what you want and giving yourself a clear path that fits your life and lights up your willpower. With SMART as your blueprint, it's like building a bridge between where you are now and where you want to be.

Stress the importance of consistency over intensity for long-term success

It's easy to get caught up in the hype of intense workouts, thinking if you're not gasping for breath by the end, then you're not doing it right. But the truth is, for most of us living regular lives with jobs, families, and to-do lists as long as our arms, consistency in our exercise routine is the real game changer. Let's talk about why.

Consistency is like the quiet best friend that supports you day in and day out, without any drama. It's showing up for your workouts, even when they're not flashy or Instagram-worthy. It's about creating a routine that sticks, one that fits into your life so seamlessly that it becomes just like brushing your teeth – something you do without a second thought.

Now, this isn't saying intensity doesn't have its place. Of course, it does. Those heart-pumping, sweat-dripping sessions have benefits. They're great when you're short on time and want to feel like you've accomplished something. But they're not everything. If you only focus on intensity, you might dread workouts skip more than you'd like, or worse, get injured. And that's not helping anyone.

Instead, think of intensity as the spice of your fitness life. It's excellent in dashes here and there, but you want it to stay on top of the dish. Your fitness journey should be sustainable, something you can keep doing next week, month, or year. And for that, you need a base of consistency.

The beauty of consistent, regular workouts is that they add up. Like coins in a piggy bank, each ten-minute walk, each set of squats, each yoga session builds on the last. You may not feel like a superhero every time, but over weeks and months, you'll see progress. You'll feel stronger, have more energy, and be fitter. That's the magic of consistency; it's quietly powerful.

Imagine you're planting a garden. You wouldn't just water your plants once with a lot of water and hope for the best. They need regular care, a little bit of water, and consistency over time. Your body is just the same. It thrives on regular attention, not just occasional floods of effort.

And here's the kicker: when you focus on being consistent, the intensity naturally follows. As you build strength and stamina with your consistent routine, you'll naturally start pushing yourself harder. You'll begin to lift heavier, run faster, or work out a bit longer. Not because you have to but because you can.

So, don't be misled by the idea that every workout has to leave you spent to count. Real success, the lasting kind, comes from showing up regularly, doing what you can, and building those fitness levels bit by bit. It's not flashy, and it's not something that'll go viral online, but it's real, and it's how you create a fitness lifestyle that lasts a lifetime. That's the secret – a consistent effort over time transforms your health and your life.

Summary

- Consistency in exercise is more beneficial for long-term success than sporadic high-intensity workouts.

- Regular, moderate exercise can fit seamlessly into daily life and become a sustainable habit, like brushing teeth.

- While intense workouts have their place, they can lead to burnout or injury if they're the sole focus.

- Consistent, low-intensity exercise accumulates benefits over time, improving strength, energy, and overall fitness without the risk of overexertion.

- Focusing on consistent workouts allows for natural exercise intensity and duration progression as the body adapts and becomes stronger.

- The key to a successful fitness journey is regularity, which leads to sustainable health improvements and a more enjoyable, integrated approach to personal fitness.

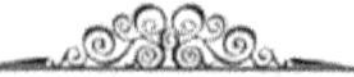

CHAPTER 3

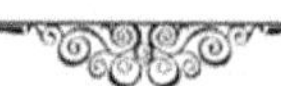

CREATING YOUR 10 -MINUTE WORKOUT PLAN

Plan your work for today and every day, and then work your plan.

Margaret Thatcher

Crafting a workout plan can sometimes feel like solving a complicated puzzle, especially when squeezing it into a jam-packed day. Yet, Margaret Thatcher's words remind us that even the busiest bees can get their fitness nectar if they've got a clear strategy. This chapter isn't about carving out hours you don't have or pushing you into a one-size-fits-all routine. Instead, it's about designing a 10-minute workout plan that molds into your life, not vice versa. Think of your workout plan as your blueprint for success. You would only build a house with a plan and should develop your fitness regime with one too. Those precious ten minutes can be enough to set the foundations for a fitter, healthier you. This chapter is going to show you how to make every minute count. We'll guide you through selecting exercises that get you the most bangs for your buck, time-wise. This isn't about leisurely pedaling on a bike while scrolling through your phone.

It's about targeted movements that engage multiple muscle groups and speed up your heart rate. We'll also talk about how to sequence your workouts for maximum effect, ensuring you're working hard and smart. Moreover, we'll dive into how to tailor these plans to fit your lifestyle. Whether you're a morning person who can sneak in a session before the day starts, take a quick lunch break, or unwind with a workout after work, we'll help you plot out the perfect ten minutes. Your workout plan should be as unique as you are, fitting into your schedule like that perfect piece of a puzzle. By the end of this chapter, you'll have a clear, concise workout plan that you can start immediately. One that doesn't demand more time than you can give but gives you all the benefits of a more extended workout session. So, let's get down to business and start building your fitness, ten minutes at a time.

Strategies for integrating workouts into daily routines

Imagine you have a piggy bank on your dresser, and every day, no matter what, you put a dime in it. It's just a dime. But day by day, that little pile of dimes grows, and before you know it, you've got a little treasure trove. That's precisely what we're doing with your ten-minute workouts. It's not about dumping hours into a gym session; it's about those consistent dimes of time that add up to a wealth of health.

Let's get real for a moment. Life is hectic. You may have kids, a job that never quits, or both. You might only have a full hour once you collapse at night. But ten minutes? That's doable. It's the time you might spend waiting for your coffee to brew or for that late Zoom meeting to start. It's just a fraction of your lunch break or a quick detour before your evening shower.

You're probably thinking, "Sure, ten minutes is short, but where do I even start?" First off, look at your typical day. Find those little pockets of time that slip by unnoticed. Maybe it's in the morning when you're waiting for everyone else to wake up. Slot in a brisk workout right there. Or perhaps you're usually scrolling through your phone during your break. Swap that out for a quick sweat session.

Then, it's all about making it as easy as possible to get moving. Keep your workout gear handy. That could mean dumbbells by your desk or workout clothes laid out the night before. The less you have to think about getting ready, the more likely you'll jump in and get moving.

And if the idea of doing the same daily routine makes you yawn, don't sweat it. Mix it up! Have a couple of different practices ready to go so you can choose your adventure. Monday might be a core-crusher, while Tuesday is all about leg power. The variety will keep your muscles guessing and your mind engaged.

Remember, the goal is to make this a no-brainer. Something you don't have to debate with yourself over. It's ten minutes, after all. You can stand on one leg for ten minutes. We won't make you do that, but you get the point. The key here is to anchor these mini workouts into your day so they become as routine as brushing your teeth.

Before long, you'll start to notice something. You'll be looking forward to these moments. Your body will crave that quick hit of activity. And like magic, those dimes of time you've been depositing will have turned into solid gold fitness gains, all without turning your life upside down to fit in a workout.

So, forget the "go hard or go home" motto. Let's make it "go smart and stay steady." You're building a habit; like that piggy bank, every little bit counts. Those ten minutes are your secret weapon, your quiet rebellion against a schedule that seems to demand everything from you. It's your claim to something invaluable—your health and well-being. And it starts in just ten minutes.

Tips on staying committed to a 10-minute daily exercise plan

Sticking to a workout plan can take time and effort. It's easy to say, "I'll just do it tomorrow," but when tomorrow rolls around, there's another excuse waiting. So, how do you break the cycle? It's all about making your 10-minute daily exercise plan as sticky as your favorite morning cereal.

First things first, you need to nail down a "why." Not just any why, but your why. Why do you want to fit these workouts into your day? Maybe you want to keep up with your kids without getting winded, or you're looking to manage stress. Your reason must be something that lights a fire in you and gets you moving, even when the couch calls your name.

Now, let's talk about your when. Everyone has a time of day when they feel most energetic. Maybe you're a morning person who loves the quiet before the world wakes up, or perhaps evenings are when you come alive. Pinpoint that time and guard it fiercely. That's your workout window.

But what happens when life throws a wrench in your plan? Maybe you oversleep, or work runs late. Here's where the magic word comes into play: flexibility— missed your morning window? Squeeze in your workout during lunch or while dinners in the oven. The point is not to let a missed moment derail your whole day.

And you've got to keep it interesting. Doing the same old routine can get boring fast. So, keep a small arsenal of exercises at your disposal. One day, you could focus on strength, another on cardio, and maybe throw some yoga to mix it up. The variety will keep boredom at bay and work different muscle groups.

Another tip? Make it social. Even if you're not into group classes, having someone to share your workout journey with can be a game-changer. Find a friend or coworker who's also into short workouts and become each other's cheerleaders. Share routines, challenge each other, and celebrate the wins together.

What about those days when motivation is in short supply? That's when your environment can save the day. Create a space just for working out, even if it's just a corner of your living room. Fill it with cues that say, "It's going time," like your sneakers, a yoga mat, or dumbbells. Make it a place you want to be.

Lastly, track your progress. It doesn't have to be a fancy fitness tracker or app. A simple calendar to mark off each day's workout will do. Seeing those entire check marks lineup is surprisingly satisfying and motivating.

The beauty of the 10-minute workout is that it's just 10 minutes. It's a short commitment, but it's a commitment nonetheless. So take it seriously, but don't be too hard on yourself. Miss a day? Shake it off. Each day is a new chance to hit that 10-minute mark. With each tick of the clock, you're building a healthier, happier you. And that's something worth committing to.

Ways to adapt workout times and types to match energy and schedules

Exercise can be like that friend who's always trying to meet up – you love them, but finding the time can be a puzzle. Ten-minute workouts? They're the quick coffee catch-ups that fit into any packed schedule. But even then, some days are unpredictable, like a deck shuffled by a magician. Here's the deal: You can make these quick workouts fit regardless of your day.

First up, know your rhythm. We all have that time when we feel like we could run a marathon or at least jog to the mailbox. Find that golden hour – or more like golden minutes – and claim it for your workout. Maybe you're a dawn patroller who can move those muscles before the rooster crows or a night owl who gets a second wind when the stars come out. It doesn't matter when; what matters is that it's your time.

Now, life can be challenging, and sometimes, your schedule will get flipped upside down. Maybe the morning got away from you, and suddenly, its bedtime, and you've not moved a muscle. Here's where you get crafty. Too tired at night? Slot in a quick session while waiting for your pasta to boil or after brushing your teeth. Who says you can't do squats while the coffee's brewing or lunges on the way to the laundry? The idea is to piggyback your workout onto something you're already doing.

Speaking of what you're already doing, let's talk about types of workouts. On days when you're feeling like a superhero, high-intensity stuff might be your jam. But then there are the days when you feel more like a sidekick – those are perfect for a low-impact routine, which gets the blood flowing without making you feel like you're climbing Mount Everest. Mix it up according to how you feel. Listen to your body; it's a smart cookie.

And hey, routines are great, but sometimes they can feel a bit like that old pair of slippers – comfortable but dull. Keep things fresh by having a few different workout options ready to go. Maybe you have a mini-circuit for when you're full of beans, a yoga flow for when you need to unwind, and a quick strength session for when you want to feel powerful. Switch it up to keep yourself interested and your body guessing.

Remember, this is your show. If your day's more jam-packed than a clown car, shorten your workout. It's better to do a super-focused five-minute session than to skip it altogether. And on those rare days when time is your friend, why not double up and go for a full twenty?

Remember it's not about being perfect. Some days, your workout will be a checkmark on your to-do list, and that's fine. On other days, you'll have to squeeze it in between meetings or while your kid's soccer practice is running over. That's fine, too. The real win is making exercise a non-negotiable part of your day, like brushing your teeth or charging your phone. Before you know it, those ten minutes will be as much a part of your routine as your morning cup of joe – simple, satisfying, and doable, no matter how hectic life gets.

Summary

- Determine the part of the day when you feel most energetic and committed to slotting in your workout, whether it's early morning, lunchtime, or evening.

- If your preferred workout time gets disrupted, find small windows throughout the day – like waiting for dinner to cook or during a break at work – to fit in quick exercise bursts.

- Match the workout intensity to your energy levels on any given day, alternating between high-intensity exercises and lower-impact activities to stay engaged without burning out.

- Mix workout routines to keep things exciting and cater to your mood and energy. This could include circuits, strength training, or even gentle stretching.

- If a day is too hectic, doing a shorter workout is okay. The aim is consistency, not perfection.

- When you have more time, extend your workout to 20 minutes or split it into two sessions to maximize benefits.

- Squeeze in exercises during routine activities, such as doing calf raises while brushing your teeth or choosing stairs over the elevator.

- Treat your workout like any other critical daily activity to ensure it gets done, fostering a habit that will stick with you in the long run.

CHAPTER 4

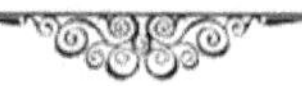

WORKOUT 1 - FULL-BODY BLAST

The key is not the will to win. Everybody has that. It is the will to prepare to win that is important.

- Bobby Knight

When it comes to exercise, sometimes less can be more. There's a saying that fits well with our fast-paced lives: Are you ready to leap into the fitness world but only have 10 minutes to spare? No problem. Chapter 5 of "10-Minute Fitness" introduces you to the "Full-Body Blast," a workout that doesn't mess around. It's short, yes, but it's also sweet in the way only a truly effective burst of exercise can be.

Imagine a workout that touches every muscle group, ignites your metabolism, and leaves you feeling surprisingly refreshed – all within the time it might take you to check your morning emails. Whether at home or on the go, the Full-Body Blast is designed to maximize your time without needing a gym total of equipment. All you need are dumbbells and a weight bench, and you'll be on your way to a firmer, more toned you.

In the coming pages, we'll break down each exercise, explaining the movements, the muscles you'll engage, and how to ensure you're getting the most out of every rep. This chapter isn't just about giving you a list of exercises; it's about starting a journey toward a healthier, more energetic life, even on a tight schedule.

Paul Cannon believes that fitness should be accessible, achievable, and, most importantly, straightforward. So, let's get started on this journey together, where your dedication to just 10 minutes can lead to surprising and utterly satisfying results.

Detailed plan for a 10-minute full-body workout

If you've ever thought you need at least an hour in a crowded gym to get a real workout, think again. A 10-minute full-body workout can do wonders, and I will show you how. No fluff, no wasted time - just straight-up exercises that hit every major muscle group, fit into your busy life and leave you feeling energized.

First, let's talk about what you need. Grab a pair of dumbbells. The weight should be heavy enough to challenge you by the last rep but not so heavy that you can't complete the set with good form. Then, find a weight bench or any sturdy surface supporting your weight. That's it - you're all set.

Now, the plan is simple. You'll spend one minute on each exercise and move quickly to the next without resting. This keeps your heart rate up, which is good for burning calories and building endurance.

Start with squats. Hold a dumbbell in each hand at your shoulders, feet shoulder-width apart. Push your hips back and lower down as if sitting in a chair, then push through your heels to stand back up. This works your legs and glutes, and holding the dumbbells also engages your arms and core.

Next up is the dumbbell bench press. Lie on the bench with a dumbbell in each hand, arms straight up over your chest. Lower the weights to your chest level and press them back up. This blasts your chest, shoulders, and triceps.

Third, go for bent-over rows. Bend at the waist, let the dumbbells hang at arm's length, and then pull them up to your sides, squeezing your shoulder blades together. This hits your upper back and biceps.

Don't rest yet—transition into the shoulder press. Please stand up, dumbbells at your shoulders, and press them straight up until your arms are extended, then lower back down. Your shoulders are working hard here, along with your upper back and core.

Half way there. It's time for dead lifts. With dumbbells in front, hinge at your hips, lower them to the ground, keep your back straight, and then stand up. This is great for your hamstrings, glutes, and lower back.

For the sixth minute, let's blast that abs with Russian twists. Sit on the floor with knees bent, lean back slightly, hold a dumbbell with both hands and twist from side to side. Your entire core is firing to keep you balanced.

Now, hit the deck for push-ups. No weights are needed here, just your body and gravity. If regular push-ups are challenging, drop to your knees - no shame. You're still working your chest, shoulders, and triceps.

For your eighth exercise, it's time for lunges. Step forward with one foot and lower your hips until both knees are bent at a 90-degree angle. Switch legs. Your legs and glutes will thank you.

On to the ninth minute with dumbbell curls. Stand with weights at your sides, palms forward, and curl the weights up to your shoulders. Your biceps are the stars now.

Finally, finish with plank rows. In a plank position, row one dumbbell up to your waist, then the other. It's tough, hitting your core, back, and arms.

And there you have it—ten exercises, one minute each, and a full-body workout that leaves no muscle untouched. Ten minutes is all it takes to challenge yourself and push toward being a fitter, more vital you. Stick with it; you'll be amazed at what these quick sessions can do for your fitness journey.

Here's a step-by-step guide to a 10-minute full-body workout. Remember, you're spending only one minute on each exercise, moving swiftly from one to the next.

1.   **Squats with Dumbbells**: Stand with feet slightly wider than shoulder-width apart. Hold a dumbbell in each hand at shoulder level. Push your hips back and lower your body until your thighs is parallel to the floor, then push back up. This targets your lower body and core.

2.   **Dumbbell Bench Press**: Lie on your back on a bench. Hold a dumbbell in each hand at chest level, palms facing forward. Push the dumbbells until your arms are straight, and then lower them back down. This exercise works on your chest, shoulders, and arms.

3.   **Bent-Over Rows**: Bend your knees slightly, bending forward at the waist while keeping your back straight. Let the dumbbells hang down. Pull the dumbbells to your side, squeezing your shoulder blades together, and then lower them back down. This targets your back and biceps.

4.   **Shoulder Press**: Stand up, holding dumbbells at shoulder height. Press them upwards until your arms are

extended overhead, and then bring them back down. This works the shoulders and engages your core.

5.   **Dumbbell Deadlifts**: Stand with feet hip-width apart, dumbbells in front of thighs. Hinge at the hips to lower the dumbbells to the ground, keeping your back flat, and then straighten back up. This hits the back of your legs and your lower back.

6.   **Russian Twists**: Sit on the ground with knees bent and lean back slightly. Hold a single dumbbell with both hands in front of you. Twist your torso to one side, then the other, engaging your oblique muscles.

7.   **Push-Ups**: Get into a plank position, hands wider than your shoulders. Lower your body until your chest nearly touches the floor then pushes back up. You can modify by dropping to your knees if necessary.

8.   **Lunges**: Stand straight, step forward with one leg, and lower your hips until both knees are bent at about a 90-degree angle. Make sure your front knee is directly above your ankle. Push back up to the starting position and repeat with the other leg.

9.   **Dumbbell Curls**: Stand with your arms at your sides, with a dumbbell in each hand. Curl the weights up to your shoulders, keeping your elbows close to your body, and then slowly lower them back down. This is for your biceps.

10.   **Plank Rows**: Hold a dumbbell in each hand on the floor in a plank position—row one dumbbell up to the side of your chest, then back down. Repeat with the other arm. This one challenges your core, back, and arms.

Take a deep breath—you've

I just completed a full-body workout in 10 minutes! Consistency is critical so that this quick blast can keep you on track toward your

The muscles worked and the benefits of each movement

Imagine squeezing a gym session into a coffee break. That's the magic of a 10-minute full-body workout. It's not about having time; it's about making time. And this quick routine is all about efficiency, hitting every major muscle group, getting your heart rate up, and boosting your metabolism.

Let's break it down, exercise by exercise:

You start with squats holding dumbbells. This isn't just a leg exercise; it's a full-body move. Your thighs and gluts power you up, your arms and shoulders work to hold the weights, and your core muscles keep you stable. It's like the Swiss Army knife of exercises—so many benefits!

The dumbbell bench press is about more than just getting more muscular arms. It also engages your chest and shoulders, pushing against gravity. As you control the dumbbells down, your muscles fine-tune the movement, which means you're working even on the way back.

Then there are the bent-over rows. This move targets the muscles you don't see in the mirror but are critical for posture—the back and biceps. As you pull those weights, think of squeezing a pencil between your shoulder blades. It's a subtle move with mighty benefits, like a shadow working hard behind the scenes.

The shoulder press comes next. It's not just for show-off muscles; it's a functional exercise. You'll thank these shoulder workouts every time you put a carry-on into the overhead bin or push your kid on the swing. It also engages your core big time. Have you ever tried pressing weights overhead without tightening your stomach? Exactly. It's a no-go.

Dumbbell deadlifts seem straightforward, but they're an all-star move. They hit the back of your legs—hello, hamstrings—and your glutes, plus they're essential for a strong lower back. And while you lift and lower those dumbbells, your core works overtime to keep your back from rounding.

Russian twists are subsequent; you're not just working your waistline while twisting. Your entire core, including those deep abdominal muscles, is firing. It's like wringing out a towel—but the towel is your midsection, and instead of water, you're shedding weakness.

Don't underestimate push-ups. They're like the old friend who has stuck with you through thick and thin. They sculpt your chest, shoulders, and triceps; when done right, they're a sneaky way to work your core, too.

The lunges are a powerhouse for lower-body strength. They're like a road trip for your legs—each works independently, driving you forward, strengthening your thighs and glutes, and improving your balance and coordination.

Dumbbell curls might seem like a vanity move, but muscular biceps are helpful for everyday lifting and pulling. And the act of controlling the weight both up and down? That's where the real magic happens because muscle control is just as important as muscle size.

Lastly, the plank row is a sneaky multitasked. It hits your arms, sure, but it also challenges the heck out of your core. Every time you row one dumbbell, your entire body has to stabilize to keep you from tipping over. It's like staying upright in a rowboat on a windy day.

These movements are more than just a way to work muscles—they're about building a body that works for you, making you more robust, agile, and equipped to handle life's physical demands. In just 10 minutes, you're not only burning calories but also building a foundation of strength, flexibility, and endurance that serves you in the long run. It's about quality, not quantity, and that's something everyone has time for.

Summary

- The workout is designed to maximize efficiency, targeting all major muscle groups within a 10-minute window.

- A compound exercise that works the thighs, glutes, arms, shoulders, and core.

- Strengthens the chest, arms, and shoulders, emphasizing movement control.

- Focuses on the back and biceps, vital for posture and stability.

- A functional exercise that engages the shoulders, arms, and core, practical for everyday activities.

- Hits the hamstrings, glutes, and lower back, involving the core for stability.

- Works the entire core region, focusing on the oblique muscles for rotational strength.

- A classic exercise that targets the chest, shoulders, triceps, and core.

- Strengthens the lower body, improves balance, and enhances coordination.

- Not just for aesthetics, they strengthen the biceps and improve muscle control.

- A challenging move that works the arms and significantly engages the core for stabilization.
- Beyond muscle work, the routine is crafted to improve overall body strength, agility, and endurance, making it ideal for a busy lifestyle.

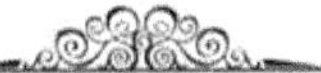

CHAPTER 5

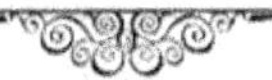

WORKOUT 2 - CHEST AND ARMS SCULPT

Strength does not come from the body. It comes from the will

— Mahatma Gandhi.

In the bustling flow of daily life, carving out time for the gym can seem like trying to move mountains. Yet, as Gandhi reminds us, where there's a will, there's a way — even if it's just ten minutes at a stretch. That's what Chapter 6, "Workout Two: Chest and Arms Sculpt," is all about. It's designed to show you how, with a pair of dumbbells and a bench, you can simultaneously strengthen your will and your body.

This chapter takes you through a focused chest and arms workout compact enough to slot into your busy schedule but potent sufficient to sculpt your muscles and enhance your upper body strength. Forget the notion that you need hours in the gym; here, every second counts.

This isn't about becoming a bodybuilder or pushing yourself to extremes. It's about intelligent, concentrated efforts that fit into your slivers of time, building your physical strength with the mental toughness that says "yes" to health, even on the busiest days.

So get ready to pick up those dumbbells. It's time to craft strength, build confidence, and sculpt your body, ten minutes at a time.

Focused 10-minute routine for the chest and biceps

Imagine you've just closed your laptop after a hectic work day, or you're about to start your morning, and you have this small window before the day's demands pull you in all directions. You think you can't possibly fit in a workout. But what if I told you that in just 10 minutes, you could fire up your chest and biceps, feel the burn, and still have time to grab a coffee before your next meeting?

This is where a sharp, focused 10-minute chest and biceps routine comes into play. It's not about long hours lifting weights; it's about making the most of your time. And you can do this right at home; no need to hustle to the gym.

Start with a quick warm-up test; getting those muscles ready is critical, even in a short workout. You could do arm circles, shoulder shrugs, and maybe a quick jog in place — to get the blood flowing.

Then, dive into the heart of your mini-workout. Begin with push-ups, the bread and butter for your chest. They don't require any equipment, and they're super effective. Do as many as you can for two minutes straight. Keep your body straight from head to heels, and push with power.

Next, if you have a set of dumbbells, grab them for bicep curls. Stand straight, weights in hand, palms facing forward, and bring the consequences to your shoulders. Keep it controlled — no swinging — and feels the tension in your biceps. Another two minutes here, and your arms should be warming up to the idea that this short burst of activity is serious business.

Now it's time for a chest press. If you have a bench, great, but the floor will do just fine. Lie down with dumbbells in your hands and press them toward the ceiling. Bring them down slowly until your elbows are below the bench or floor, then push back up. Spend two minutes here, and remember to breathe.

Wait to take a breather; keep the pace up with hammer curls for the biceps. Hold the dumbbells with your palms facing each other and curl this time. This variation hits different parts of your biceps and forearms. Again, give it a solid two minutes of your ten-minute cap.

To finish, alternate between push-ups and curls, one minute each, to completely exhaust the muscles. You're creating a circuit that maximizes your effort in a minimum amount of time.

By the time you're done, your chest and biceps will have had a workout intense enough to count, and you'll still have 23 hours and 50 minutes left in your day to do everything else. It's not about the length of time but the quality and intensity you pack into it. And there, in the reflection of your computer screen or window, you'll see the person who just made a powerful choice for their health, all in the space of a quick coffee break. Now, take on the rest of your day with the same vigor you just pumped into that 10-minute burst of fitness.

Tips and dumbbell technique guidance

Imagine squeezing in a workout between your endless to-dos. You've only got dumbbells and a sliver of time, but that's enough. Getting your form right in an activity, especially when handling weights, is like hitting the bullseye in archery — it makes all the difference. And the best part it's not complicated.

When you're doing bicep curls, it's not just an up-and-down movement. Stand up straight, and keep those elbows close to your body like glued to your ribs. When you lift, it's just your forearm moving, nothing else. Those are cheats, no swinging, no leaning back, and we're not here for that. Lift the weight smoothly up to your shoulder, pause for a second, and then lower it down just as slowly. That's where the magic happens, in the slow release, not just the lift.

And it's pretty similar to hammer curls, but think about holding a hammer — that's how your hands should be facing. This slight twist in the wrist works different muscles and ads to your arm strength in ways a regular curl doesn't. It's the small changes that bring significant results.

Now, let's talk about the chest press. If you're lying on the floor, that's cool — it's an excellent way to ensure you don't drop your elbows too low. When pressing those dumbbells, push them straight up to the ceiling and bring them down until your elbows touch the floor gently. You can go lower on a bench, but never let your elbows drop below shoulder level. That's how you keep your shoulders safe.

Here's a tip: When you push up, imagine you're trying to make the dumbbells meet at the top without clanging them together. This mental image helps engage the chest muscles even more.

And form isn't just about how you move; it's about how you breathe. Inhale when you're bringing the weights down, and exhale when you're exerting force, like lifting the dumbbells during the bicep curl or pressing them up in the chest press. This breathing technique gives you power and keeps you from getting dizzy.

You might wonder if you're doing it right. Here's a hint: if you can chat about your day or plan dinner during your reps, you should increase the weight or focus more on your technique. You should be able to breathe but not belt out your favorite song.

Remember, those dumbbells are tools, and you're the craftsman. Every lift, curl, and press is a stroke of art on the canvas of fitness. Your muscles respond to how well you use these tools, and you're sculpting a more muscular you with each correct move.

In those ten minutes, with just the right moves and technique, you're not just passing time but building strength. And when it's done, you step back into your day not just feeling more alive but armed with the quiet confidence of someone who knows they're taking care of their body.

How to modify exercises for different fitness levels

Getting fit isn't a one-size-fits-all journey. Whether you're just starting or you've been at this fitness game for a while, your exercises should match your fitness level. That's the beauty of working out; you can tweak it to challenge you just enough without pushing you over the edge.

So, you're staring at an exercise routine, and it's got push-ups. If you're new to this, a full push-up is like lifting a mountain with your pinky finger. No problem. You can start with wall push-ups, standing up, and pushing away from the wall. It's gentler, but you're still working those muscles. Ready for a bit more? Try knee push-ups on the ground. It's like a push-up, but your knees are your base, not your toes. And when you feel like a champ, go for the full push-up, your body straight as a ruler and your hands powering you up and down.

Now, let's say squats are up next. If you've never done one, don't just drop down and hope for the best. You can start by sitting down and standing up from a chair. It's a squat without the fear of not being able to get up. Feel good about those? Step away from the chair and squat like you're about to sit in it, but stop just before you touch it, then stand back up. And if you're thinking, "I've got this," then go ahead and squat with no chair behind you, as if you're sitting in an invisible chair. Keep that back straight, and don't let your knees creep over your toes.

Lunges are following, and they're great for your legs. But they can be tricky. Start with a small step forward, not too far, just enough to bend that knee. As you get the hang of it, increase the step until you can lower your back knee toward the ground without letting it touch. And if you're already lunging like a pro, grab some weights and add a little extra challenge as you step forward.

What about cardio, though? If running isn't your thing yet, brisk walking is a solid start. Walking faster or finding a hill to conquer can get your heart rate up. Jogging can come next, even if it's just for a few minutes at a time. And when you're ready to run full-on, set your pace and knock out those sprints.

The key is to listen to your body. It knows when you can push a little harder or when you need to dial it back. The goal is to make progress, not to prove a point. And progress looks different for everyone. It's not about keeping up with the person next to you at the gym or someone's highlight reel on social media. It's about being a little better than you were yesterday.

So, modify as you need, and remember that every modified move is still a move toward your fitness goals. Your workout is yours, and it's there to make you stronger, not to knock you down. Keep at it, and you'll find your strength building, your confidence growing, and your exercises evolving to match the fantastic work you're putting in.

Summary

- The chapter begins with an overview of the importance of strengthening the upper body for functional and aesthetic purposes.
- It outlines a time-efficient 10-minute workout to sculpt the chest and arm muscles.
- The chapter details a selection of exercises targeting the pectorals, biceps, triceps, and shoulders, emphasizing the effectiveness of each movement for muscle development.
- Key points on maintaining correct form and technique during exercises are provided to maximize gains and reduce the risk of injury.
- Strategies for progressing the exercises to keep challenging the muscles as they grow stronger and adaptations for various fitness levels are discussed.
- Suggestions are made on combining this routine with other workouts from the book for a more comprehensive fitness regimen.

- The chapter suggests using minimal equipment, like dumbbells, to add resistance to the workout, with alternative options for those without access to equipment.

- Tips on recovery and the importance of rest between workouts targeting the same muscle groups are provided to ensure proper muscle recovery and growth.

- The chapter concludes with motivational advice on staying consistent with the chest and arms sculpt routine for best results.

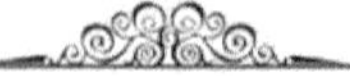

CHAPTER 6

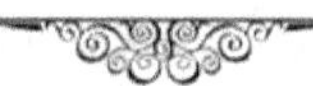

WORKOUT 3 - CORE STRENGTHENING CIRCUIT

Strength does not come from physical capacity. It comes from an indomitable will.

Mahatma Gandhi

Strong core muscles are at the heart of every movement you make. In Chapter 7, titled "Workout Three: Core Strengthening Circuit," the focus shifts to the powerhouse of the body—the core. The core is not just about having a well-defined abdomen; it's the central link connecting your upper and lower bodies. A robust and resilient spirit is essential for stability and strength in everyday activities and complex exercises. This chapter dives into a circuit workout that's crafted to enhance the strength and endurance of your core muscles within a time-efficient, 10-minute framework. Whether you're a busy professional, a parent juggling multiple tasks, or someone simply looking to improve their fitness without spending hours at the gym, this workout is designed to fit into your schedule. You will discover exercises that challenge every part of your core, including the deep abdominal muscles, the obliques, and the lower back. The guidance provided will ensure that you can perform each exercise with proper form, which is crucial for preventing injuries and reaping the full benefits of the workout.

Embrace the challenge, and let this core strengthening circuit be a pivotal part of your fitness journey, offering a practical solution to building a strong, supple, and functional core that supports your body through all walks of life.

A quick, intense core workout routine

Imagine slipping in a workout those fires up your core in 10 minutes. That's less time than it takes to finish your morning coffee. This chapter isn't about leisurely sit-ups with breaks to check messages. It's about igniting a core workout that's fast, furious, and to the point.

First, picture this: You've got 10 minutes. What can you do in that time? You can crank the intensity and challenge every muscle between your shoulders and hips. The beauty of a core circuit is that it doesn't need any fancy equipment or a gym membership—just a bit of floor space and a willingness to push you.

The routine starts with planks, but not just any planks. You will cycle through side planks and regular planks to hit every angle. Picture your body as a straight line from head to heels, muscles tight as a drum. You'll hold each plank for 30 seconds, but it'll feel longer because you're keeping your body rigid, your core screaming.

Next, you're onto crunches, but with a twist. Bicycle crunches mix leg movement and a torso twist, sparking life into the oblique's side muscles. Each knee comes up to meet the opposite elbow, and you'll keep the pace brisk. It's about quality, not just speed, feeling each muscle work as you switch sides.

Then, without wasting a second, it's on to the Russian twists. Sitting up with knees bent, you lean back just enough to feel your abs kick in. With hands together, you'll twist side to side. This isn't a gentle swaying but a deliberate, controlled twist, working the core to its full potential.

And when you think you can't go on, flip over for the Superman pose. Lying face down, you'll lift your arms and legs, holding the position, your back, and glutes working hard. It's a hero's move, and though no one's watching, you'll feel like a champion holding it as long as you can.

Finally, finish with mountain climbers. Fast feet drive your workout home, bringing the heart rate up, the sweat pouring down, and your breath to heavy pants. It's the climax of your 10-minute epic, the full-body shake-up that leaves no doubt you've worked every inch of your core.

And there you have it. In the time it takes to scroll through your social media feed, you've blasted through a core routine that some wouldn't manage in an hour. It's intense, sure, but it's also over before you know it, leaving you pumped and ready to tackle whatever comes next in your day. This is more than just a workout; it's a statement that you don't need to clear your schedule to keep fit. All you need is a short burst of undiluted effort and the commitment to make every minute count.

Include instructions for exercises that target the entire core

Diving into a core workout can seem like a trip to the dentist – necessary but not always pleasant. Yet, the truth is, a strong core sets you up for almost every activity you do, whether it's bending down to tie a shoe or hitting a new squat personal best. And guess what? You can fire up your core in 10 minutes with simple, swift, and super-effective exercises.

Kick things off with the classic plank. It's like the bread and butter of core exercises – basic but powerful. Get down on the floor on your elbows and toes, keep your back flat, and hold. Your body should form a straight line from your shoulders to your ankles. Engage your abs as if bracing for a punch in the gut. Hold it for 30 seconds. It's tough but thinks about something that makes you smile to pass the time.

Next up, give side planks a go. They're like the cousin of the plank but with a twist. Lie on your side, prop yourself on one elbow, and stack your feet. Then, lift your hips until your body makes a diagonal line from head to feet. Hold for 30 seconds on each side. Imagine a wall in front and behind you – you want to stay flat enough to fit between them.

Don't let up now; switch to bicycle crunches. Lie on your back, hands behind your head, and lift your shoulders. Bring your right elbow to your left knee, then switch. It's like pedaling a bike upside-down—and just as fun when you get into the rhythm.

After that, take a second to lie flat – enjoy it; it's part of the workout. Then, go into leg raises. Lift your legs straight up, and then lower them slowly just before touching the floor. Lift them again. This isn't a race; it's gradually just before touching abs working.

Follow it with Russian twists. Sit up, knees bent, and lean back slightly. Twist to touch the floor beside you, alternating sides. No need to rush; pretend you're wringing out a wet towel with your torso – get every last drop out.

Finish with mountain climbers. Get into a push-up position, and then run your knees into your chest, one at a time, like you're scaling the steepest hill. It's like a sprint for your core, so push the pace, but remember, form is king.

Remember, you're not trying to win a medal here. The goal is to stay moving, keep that core engaged, and power through until the end. Each exercise targets a different part of your core, from the six-pack abs at the front to the often-neglected muscles wrapping around your sides and back.

By the time your 10 minutes are up, you'll have worked every angle of your core. And here's the kicker – you'll feel stronger in everything you do because a solid body is the foundation of all strength. Plus, you'll carry yourself a little taller, knowing you've taken another step toward being your strongest self, and all it took was 10 minutes of pure determination.

The importance of core strength for overall fitness

When you hear the word "core," you might think of abs that are all about looking good on the beach, but it's so much more than that. Core strength is a big deal for your body and critical player in all your moves. It's not just about crunches and planks; your core is the center of your body's power, like the sturdy tree trunk that holds everything together.

Think of your core muscles as the boss of your body. They're in charge of keeping you stable and ensuring everything else can do its job right. Whether you're picking up a heavy box, reaching to grab something off a high shelf, or even sitting at your desk, your core is working overtime to keep you balanced and upright.

Strong core muscles are like the world's best bodyguard for your spine. They help you stand up straight, protect your back from injury, and give you the power to lift, twist, and move. Without a strong core, every time you lift something heavy or turn it to look behind you, you're risking a back strain or worse.

But core strength isn't just for lifting weights or doing fancy yoga poses. It's about everyday life. Have you ever felt your back ache after a long car ride? Or you've noticed your posture slouched after sitting for too long. That's your core muscles telling you they need a workout.

Here's the thing: when your core is strong, you're like a well-built house. Everything else – your arms, legs, and brain – works well. Good core strength can make you a better runner because your midsection holds your pelvis, hips, and lower back in alignment, meaning less energy is wasted with every step. If you play sports, a strong core can give you the balance to take a hit and keep going or the power to nail that killer serve in tennis.

Even if you're not into sports, a beefy core can make daily tasks a walk in the park. Groceries feel lighter, climbing stairs becomes more accessible, and that tired feeling at the end of the day? It could take a hike because a robust core keeps you efficient and less prone to fatigue.

And here's a fun fact: working on your core can improve your breathing. Yep, because those muscles are close buddies with your diaphragm – the force that helps you inhale and exhale. So, a solid core means every breath you take is more powerful. It's like giving your body a mini spa treatment with every inhale.

In a nutshell, your core is the unsung hero of your body's fitness saga. It's not about getting a six-pack for selfies – it's about making life easier, safer, and even more fun. Core strength puts the "able" in "capable," so every time you work on it, you invest in a fitter future for yourself. So give those core muscles the love they deserve, and they'll pay you back with strength, stability, and stamina to tackle whatever life throws your way.

Summary

- Core strength is fundamental for overall body stability and strength, not just for aesthetic abs.
- The core muscles act as the body's stabilizers in nearly every movement and are essential for balance and posture.
- A strong core is crucial for protecting the spine and preventing back pain and injuries.
- Core fitness enhances daily activities, making routine tasks easier and reducing fatigue.
- Good core strength supports other fitness activities, like running and sports, by maintaining proper alignment and efficiency.
- Strong core muscles also contribute to better breathing by supporting the diaphragm.
- Developing core strength is an investment in long-term health and fitness, beyond just improving physical appearance.
- Regular core workouts lead to improved performance in physical activities, both in sports and day-to-day life.

- Building core strength ensures a solid foundation for the body, much like a strong trunk is essential for a tree's stability and growth.
- Emphasizing core training in a workout regimen can have far-reaching benefits for overall fitness and well-being.

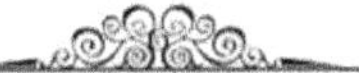

CHAPTER 7

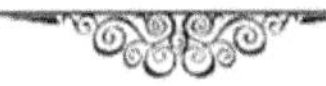

WORKOUT 4 - POWER LEGS

When you're on a long run, and your legs are tired and your mind is spent, that's when it gets tough.

Kathrine Switzer

But it's also where you find your strength. In Chapter 8, titled "Workout Four: Power Legs," we deeply dive into how you can create strength in your lower body, even when your schedule is tight. Your legs are:

- Your foundation.
- Carrying you through your day.
- Step by step.
- Providing the power behind your movements.

A 10-minute leg workout might not make a big difference, but you'd be surprised how effective it can be when it's all about targeting the right muscles with the right moves.

This chapter isn't just about getting more muscular legs. It's about enhancing your overall stamina, improving your balance, and giving you a burst of energy that lasts all day. With a focus on power, you'll learn exercises that engage every muscle in your legs, from your calves to your glutes. We've tailored these workouts to fit into your life so that you can do them at home, in the park, or even in a small space at the office.

Power legs are more than just muscle; they're about the strength to push through barriers and the endurance to keep going when it gets tricky. Let's get ready to build some serious muscle in those legs, ten minutes at a time.

A 10-minute workout focused on leg strength and endurance

You have ten minutes. In that brief pocket, you could scroll through social media, wait for your coffee to brew, or power up your legs with a workout that leaves you buzzing all day.

Here's how to turn a mere 600 seconds into a solid leg session. Picture yourself in your workout gear, ready to transform those ten minutes into a leg-strengthening blitz. You're going to hit the start button on your timer and dive straight into squats without any fuss. These are your bread and butter – simple, no equipment needed, and they target almost every muscle in your lower body. Keep the form tight and the pace steady. You'll do as many as you can in a minute.

Next up, lunges. Alternate legs and step forward, dropping your hips down to where your front thigh is parallel to the floor. That burn you feel? Your quads, glutes, and hamstrings are stepping up to the plate—another minute ticks by.

Let's get your heart pumping—it's time for some high knees. Push the pace, get those knees up, and pump your arms. This isn't just good for strength; it's a mini cardio session. One minute of high knees, and you'll feel the heat rise.

Have you got a step or a sturdy box? Step-ups are next. They're like lunges but with an added challenge. You'll drive up through your heel, activating the muscles in your legs even more. Alternate legs, keep your chest up and your eyes forward. One minute, and you're halfway through.

Take a quick breath. Now, let's hit the floor for some glute bridges. Heels down, hips up, squeeze those glutes at the top. It's a powerhouse move for your backside, ensuring every part of your legs gets the attention they deserve.

You're five minutes in. Are you feeling good? Let's keep rolling. Side lunges come next. They target the inner and outer thighs, which often get less love during workouts. Keep it smooth, side to side, stretching and strengthening as you go.

It's time to revisit squats, but with a twist – literally. Add a twist towards the lifted knee as you come up from each squat. Engage that abs, and feel the legs working. This isn't just a leg workout; you're getting an entire lower body revamp.

The final two minutes are a downhill run. Start with calf raises. Up and down on your toes, you are feeling the burn in the muscles that keep you balanced and strong on your feet. And to finish? A static squat hold. Drop down, hold low, and stay there. It's tough, it's intense, and as the final seconds tick down, you'll know you're finishing strong.

Ten minutes on the clock, and you're done. Your legs are woken up and energized, and that post-workout satisfaction sets in. You've pushed, pulled, and powered up every part of your lower body in less time than it takes to clear your morning emails. Now, take on the day with legs feeling like well-oiled machines, ready for anything.

Exercise variations for different intensity levels

Exercising is like adding a pinch of magic to your day. It can turn your mood around, boost your energy, and make you feel like you've achieved something big, even before breakfast. But everyone's different. Some of us can jump into a workout like a dolphin into the ocean, while others need to wade in slowly, like easing into a hot bath. So, here's the scoop on how to tweak your exercises so they fit you just right.

Let's take squats, for example. If you feel like Superman or Wonder Woman, you can jump into jump squats. Bend those knees, send your hips back, and then spring into the air like you're reaching for the stars. But if you're not up for jumping, no problem. Keep your feet planted firmly on the ground, squat down low, and rise on your toes. You're still getting that strength work in at a pace that suits you.

Lunges are another move that can be turned up or dialed down. If you've got energy to burn, try a lunge with a hop. Step forward into your lunge, then add a little dance as you switch legs. Feeling more like keeping it chill? Step back into reverse lunges. You'll still work those muscles without the extra impact.

High knees can be a blast. They get your heart racing and legs pumping. But let's say you're not feeling the need for speed. March is in place instead. Lift those knees high, one at a time, with purpose and power. You're moving, you're grooving, and you're keeping it at your level.

Have you got a step or a box for step-ups? If you're ready to rock, add a knee lift at the top of each step-up to challenge your balance and work your core. Step up and down in a smooth, steady rhythm if that's too much jazz for you today. You're still winning.

Glute bridges can be spiced up by adding a march. Lift into your bridge, then march your feet one at a time, keeping those hips up. Want to keep it simple? Stay with the classic bridge, pressing up and down, squeezing those glutes every time.

Side lunges can get an upgrade, too. Slide into your side lunge, then sweep the trailing leg into a sidekick, but if that sounds too much, step side to side, bending one knee and then the other, getting deep into the stretch and the strength of the move.

And for those calf raises, try them on one leg at a time if you're eager to push it. If you're keeping it mellow, do both feet together, rising and lowering, feeling solid and steady.

As for that squat hold at the end, if you're all about that burn, hold a weight at your chest to add an extra challenge. If not, just your body weight is perfect. Sink, hold on, and breathe through it. You're building strength no matter what.

Exercises are like clothes; they should fit you as you are today. Some days, you're all about that high-energy, high-intensity life, and other days, not so much. Either way, you're doing something great for yourself. And remember, whether you're taking it easy or going hard, you're lapping everyone on the couch. Keep moving, keep smiling, and make your workout your own.

The importance of leg workouts for metabolic health

Imagine you've got a car, a nice one. You'd want to make sure it runs smoothly. You'd check the oil, inflate the tires, and fill it with good gas. Well, think of your legs as the wheels of your body's car. The system runs better if they're strong and in good shape. This is about more than just looking fit or being able to jump higher or run faster. Working on your legs is a big deal for metabolic health, like the behind-the-scenes of how your body uses energy.

Your legs are packed with some of your body's biggest and most powerful muscles. When you get those muscles moving, it's like putting your metabolism on a treadmill; it has to start running. This means you burn more calories, not just when you're working out but even after, when you're chilling on the sofa or at your desk.

It's like having a car that keeps burning fuel efficiently, even at a red light.

Now, why is this so important? Because good metabolic health keeps the sugar and fat levels in your blood just right. When these levels are off, it can lead to all sorts of trouble, like diabetes or heart disease. If you put the wrong gas in your car or never changed the oil, things would go wrong under the hood.

But when you do leg workouts, you're keeping everything tuned up. Your body gets better at dealing with sugar, which means less of it hangs around in your blood, and that's a big win for your health. Plus, leg workouts can improve how your body handles insulin, which helps your body use sugar. Think of insulin as a key that unlocks your cells to use sugar as fuel. When your cells are open and working right, you don't need as much insulin floating around, which is good.

Another cool thing is that leg workouts can help you with fat, especially the kind that's not good for you, like belly fat. It's like having a unique feature in your car that helps it burn off lousy fuel before it clogs up the system. Focusing on your legs, you're helping to keep your weight in check and prevent fat from building up where it shouldn't.

And remember the bones and joints. Working on your legs keeps them strong, too. It's like making sure your car's frame is solid to handle bumpy roads without falling apart. Plus, if your legs are strong, they can take the pressure off your knees and hips, which mean those parts, will last longer and work better.

In short, leg workouts are about way more than just muscles. They help your whole body stay healthy, calm metabolism, and prevent many health problems. So, next time you're thinking about skipping leg day, remember that it's like giving your body's car a premium service. It's worth it to keep everything running right.

Summary

- Leg muscles are among the largest in the body, so working them out can significantly boost your metabolism.
- Regular leg workouts enhance calorie burn during and after exercise, contributing to better energy use even when not working out.

- Improving leg strength helps regulate blood sugar and fat levels, crucial for preventing metabolic diseases like diabetes and heart disease.

- Leg exercises improve insulin sensitivity, meaning your body requires less insulin to process sugar, reducing the risk of insulin resistance.

- Targeted leg workouts can help manage and reduce unhealthy fat deposits, such as visceral fat around the abdomen.

- Strengthening leg muscles supports bone health, reducing the risk of fractures and osteoporosis.

- Strong legs take pressure off joints, particularly in the knees and hips, potentially reducing the risk of joint-related issues and improving overall body mechanics.

- Consistent leg workouts contribute to overall weight management, essential for maintaining good metabolic health.

- Leg strength is fundamental for fitness performance and everyday activities, enhancing mobility and stability.

- Incorporating leg workouts into your routine is a proactive step toward long-term health and well-being, akin to regular maintenance of a well-functioning vehicle.

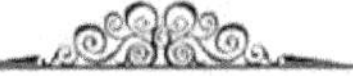

CHAPTER 8

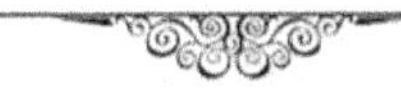

WORKOUT 5 - TOTAL BALANCE

Balance is not something you find; it's something you create,

Jana Kingsford

Takes this concept into physical health, emphasizing how a balanced body can lead to a balanced life. This chapter will guide you through the essentials of building a workout routine that doesn't just focus on strength or endurance but ensures that your body maintains equilibrium, flexibility, and coordination.

As we'll explore, balance is a critical component of overall fitness. The unsung hero allows you to stand, walk, and move with grace and efficiency. But it's often overlooked in typical training programs. This chapter addresses that gap, laying out a workout designed to challenge and improve your body's ability to balance. You'll learn about exercises that are not only about the exertion of muscles but also about the control and stabilization that come from a well-harmonized body. Through carefully selected movements, this chapter will show you how to integrate balance training into your daily regimen, ultimately enhancing your physical abilities and preventing injuries. So, get ready to discover the power of balance in your workout routine and how it can transform how you move through life.

Combine previous exercises into a balanced routine

Regarding fitness, it's not just about going hard on the treadmill or lifting heavy weights. It's about crafting a routine that touches every aspect of physical health. This is where the magic of a balanced practice comes into play. A flat performance pulls together different elements of fitness – strength, endurance, flexibility, and balance – to create a comprehensive approach to your well-being.

Think about your fitness routine as a meal. Just as you need a bit of everything on your plate to meet all your nutritional needs, your workout should include a variety of exercises to keep your body in top shape. Start with a warm-up, the appetizer, which preps your body for what's to come. Then, move on to the main course, a mix of strength training involving push-ups or lunges and endurance exercises like quick sprints or jump rope to get your heart rate up. Finally, wind down with the dessert - stretching and balance exercises that help cool down your body and improve your flexibility.

Mixing exercises from previous workouts can be like putting together a greatest hits album. You take the star exercises that work your arms, legs, chest, and core and weave them into a routine that hits every note perfectly. One minute, you could be doing squats to work on your leg strength, and the next, holding a plank to build core stability. Throw in some bicep curls with dumbbells, and you're working on those arms, too.

It's important to remember that balance isn't just standing on one foot; it's about distributing exercise evenly across your body. You don't want to overdo it with the arms and neglect the legs, or vice versa. It's like walking a tightrope; you must stay centered to avoid falling off. And that's precisely what you're doing with a balanced routine - keeping your fitness journey centered and aligned.

You want to aim for symmetry in your workouts. If you do a push exercise, like push-ups, balance it with a pull exercise, like rows. This symmetry ensures that you're not just working on one set of muscles but engaging the opposite muscles. This helps reduce the risk of injury and improves overall muscle function.

In creating your balanced routine, consider your available time and energy levels. Some days, you may have more time and energy to put into your workout, while other days, you might need something quick and less intense. The beauty of a balanced routine is that it can be adjusted to fit your day without skimping on the benefits.

Remember, a balanced routine is not set in stone. You can switch up the exercises, the order, and the intensity to fit your needs and to keep things interesting. The goal is to work out smart, not just hard. By combining different exercises into a well-rounded routine, you'll not only improve in areas like strength and endurance, but you'll also become more adept at maintaining your body's balance, both in your workouts and in your everyday life.

Focus on exercises that promote stability and muscle coordination

When we talk about getting stronger and fitter, it's easy to think it's all about how much you can bench press or how many miles you can run. But there's a secret ingredient in the fitness recipe that often gets overlooked: stability and muscle coordination. They're the unsung heroes that make all those lifts and sprints possible.

To focus on these critical areas, you don't need to be flipping tires or climbing ropes (unless you want to, of course). You can start with something as simple as standing on one leg. Sounds too easy? Try doing it with your eyes closed, and you'll notice how your muscles twitch and work to keep you upright. This is where you begin to understand stability. Your body is a complex system where everything is connected. By challenging your balance, you're giving a heads-up to those small, deep muscles that need to wake up and keep you steady.

Then, bring in exercises that demand your muscles to play nice together – we're discussing coordination. Think about a single-leg deadlift. You're not just picking something up; you're telling one leg to hold you steady while the other lifts behind you, your arms to control the weight, and your back to stay straight. It's like conducting an orchestra where your body is the symphony, and every movement is a note that needs to be in harmony with the others.

Let's remember those planks. They're not just a trendy Instagram pose but a full-body workout. Planks make your core act like a pillar, supporting your whole body, and at the same time, they ask your arms and legs to join in on the effort. The longer you hold, the more you'll feel every muscle working together, building that stability and coordination like a fortress.

We also have exercises like lunges and squats, oldies, and goodies that build strength and demand stability and muscle coordination. When you lower yourself in a squat, you're not just working your thighs; you're controlling the movement with your hips, knees, and ankles, all while keeping that back straight and core tight.

Another star is the medicine ball pass. Tossing a weighted ball might seem straightforward, but it's a ballet of muscle coordination. You're catching, balancing, and throwing while ensuring you don't topple over. It's not just your arms working here; your whole body has to harmonize to get that ball where it needs to go.

Now, this is about more than mastering each exercise right away. It's about growing more robust step by step. As you practice, your stability and coordination will get better. And the next thing you know, you're walking straighter, lifting heavier, and feeling steadier on your feet. This isn't just good for gym time; it's great for life. When you're stable and coordinated, you move better, are less likely to fall or get hurt and feel more confident in your skin.

So next time you work out, remember it's not just about pounding the pavement or lifting steel. It's about the quiet work of stability and muscle coordination, the unsung heroes that bring your fitness game together. They're the foundation for everything you do, whether on the field, in the gym, or just carrying groceries home.

By focusing on these, you're not just building a body that looks strong but a solid body from the inside out.

How balanced workouts contribute to overall fitness?

Picture your fitness routine as a team sport where every player has a crucial role. In this game, a balanced workout is your all-star player because it ensures that no part of your body is left behind. A balanced routine is the secret sauce that boosts your overall fitness, and here's how it all comes together.

Think about those days when you've got a spring in your step and feel top-notch. Chances are, it's not just because you did a bunch of arm curls or ran a few miles. It's probably because your whole body feels good, strong, and ready to take on whatever comes your way. That's what a balanced workout does for you. It's not just about making one part of your body super solid or flexible; it's about getting everything in on the action so you can feel great from head to toe.

Now, let's get down to the nitty-gritty. A balanced workout touches on a bit of everything. It's like making a smoothie and ensuring you have some greens, fruits, protein, and a little fat. For your body, this means some cardio for heart health, strength training for muscle building, flexibility exercises to keep you limber, and balance drills to keep you steady on your feet. Mixing it all up gives you a well-rounded fitness regime that helps every part of you.

Let's not forget that mixing things up keeps boredom at bay. Doing the same thing over and over can make your workout feel like a chore. But when you have a variety in your routine, you're always on your toes, eager to see what's next. This keeps your gym time fresh and exciting, making you more likely to stick with it.

A balanced routine also means you're less likely to get injured. If you only work on your upper body, you might have solid arms but weak legs. That's like having a chair with uneven legs; it's bound to wobble and possibly crash. But when you strengthen your whole body, you build a sturdy base that can handle more without breaking down.

And here's the kicker: when you work out your whole body, you strengthen in ways that matter for real life. You're not just training to look good in a tank top or running in straight lines; you're preparing to carry heavy groceries, sprinting to catch a bus, or lifting your toddler without throwing your back out. It's about making your everyday life smoother and more accessible.

In essence, a balanced workout is your ticket to a fit body and a capable one. It's about being ready for a spontaneous dance-off, a surprise hike invitation, or an impromptu soccer game with friends. It's fitness that prepares you for life's surprises and helps you live it to the fullest.

So, when you plan your fitness routine, think of it as crafting a well-balanced meal for your body that nourishes every part and leaves you feeling satisfied, strong, and unstoppable. That's the real gold of a balanced workout; fitness fits into your life, making every day a little better, more robust, and much more fun.

Summary

- A balanced workout includes cardio, strength, flexibility, and balance exercises for overall health.

- Various exercises keep the routine engaging and maintain an interest in continuing the workout regimen.

- Evenly working all muscle groups prevents imbalances and reduces the likelihood of injuries.

- Balanced training enhances day-to-day functionality, making everyday activities more accessible and less strenuous.

- The diversity of a balanced routine keeps motivation high, aiding in a long-term commitment to fitness.

- This approach builds strength across the body, ensuring no muscle group is neglected.

- A balanced workout can be adjusted to fit different fitness levels and goals, making it universally applicable.

- Incorporating stability and coordination exercises improves body control and physical performance.

- Completing varied workouts can provide a mental uplift through a sense of achievement and physical improvement.

- Balanced workouts are designed not just for fitness but to enhance the quality of life, making physical activity a pleasurable and integral part of daily living.

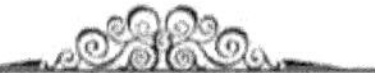

CHAPTER 9

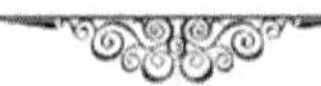

FROM MINUTES TO MOMENTUM

Consistency is not perfection; it simply refuses to give up.

– Anonymous.

Building a habit, especially one related to fitness, is like planting a garden. It begins with the simple act of sowing seeds—or, in fitness terms, starting with short, manageable workouts. Chapter 10, "From Minutes to Momentum," dives into the concept that these bite-sized commitments to your health are the starting point for something much more significant. Just as a seedling doesn't sprout into a tree overnight, the journey from a ten-minute workout to a consistent fitness routine doesn't happen instantly. It requires patience, persistence, and a bit of sweat.

This chapter is about growth. It's about how those ten-minute blocks can stack up to create a sturdy foundation for a lifelong fitness journey. It'll talk about how starting small doesn't mean staying small and how, over time, your short workouts can evolve into a momentum that powers you through more significant challenges and towards more considerable achievements. The focus isn't just on what you're doing today but on where these actions will take you tomorrow, next month, and in the years to come.

Short workouts into a consistent routine

You've got a ten-minute workout in your pocket. It's short, it's sweet, and it's all yours. You can squeeze it in before breakfast, on your lunch break, or even after a long day when you feel like doing nothing. But here's the secret sauce – those ten minutes? They're a gold mine for your health and well-being.

Now, I get it. You might think, "What will ten minutes do for me?" Well, it's not just about those ten minutes; it's about making them a regular part of your day. It's about creating a habit that sticks, and here's the thing – patterns have this funny way of snowballing. Do something for long enough, and before you know it, it's part of your routine, as normal as brushing your teeth or checking your phone.

So, how do you go from occasionally dabbling in ten-minute workouts to making them a non-negotiable part of your day? It starts with commitment. You decide that no matter what, you will do your exercise. And here's where it gets good – once you start doing it daily, it gets easier. Your body starts to crave the movement, your mind starts to rely on the break, and suddenly, it's not something you have to do; it's something you want to do.

But let's keep it accurate. Some days are going to be more challenging than others. There'll be mornings when your bed is too cozy or evenings when your couch is too comfy. That's when you need to remind yourself why you started. It could be to feel stronger, to have more energy, to sleep better, or to chase after your kids without getting winded. Your 'why' is your power. It gets you moving when everything else tells you to stay put.

Once those ten-minute workouts become a staple, something extraordinary happens. You start to notice changes – maybe your jeans fit better, you can carry more groceries, or you're not out of breath when you climb stairs. And as you notice these changes, you'll want to push for more. Maybe add another five minutes, try a new exercise, or increase the intensity. Before you know it, you're not just working out for ten minutes; you're living a more active lifestyle.

The beauty of turning short workouts into a consistent routine is that it's not about overhauling your life but enhancing it. It's about taking your time and making it work for you. It's about proving you can stick to something and watch it grow. And let's face it, there's something incredibly satisfying about that.

So, give yourself a pat on the back for every ten-minute workout you do because every single one is a step towards a healthier, happier you. Remember, fitness isn't a sprint; it's a marathon. And every minute you spend working out builds a more substantial, more resilient body and mind. Those ten minutes? They're not just part of your day but the building blocks of a vibrant, energetic life. Keep stacking them up, watch your momentum build, and enjoy where it takes you.

How to increase workout duration progressively?

When you're building fitness, increasing your workout time can sometimes feel as daunting as scaling a mountain. But it doesn't have to be. Incremental changes are your best friend here, and they can lead to impressive progress over time.

First off, think of your current exercise routine as your home base. This is where you're comfortable, but it's also your launch pad for what's next. Consider adding just a minute or two to your weekly workout to step it up. It's such a small change that you'll hardly notice it day-to-day, but over a month, you're already working out ten minutes longer. It's a game of patience and consistency.

Now, imagine you're at a stage where your ten-minute workouts are breezing by. This is where you get to play a bit. Sprinkle in an extra set of your favorite exercises, or add a new move to keep things interesting. This upsets your time and keeps your muscles guessing, which is excellent for your fitness.

Speaking of mixing it up, how about tweaking the intensity? If you've been walking, throw brisk walking or jogging in some intervals. If you're doing body-weight exercises, speed them up or add a jump. It's not just about adding time; it's about making the time you have more effective.

The trick is to do just what is necessary. If you push too hard too fast, you risk burnout or injury. So listen to your body. It's okay to take it slow. It's okay to have days where you stick to your usual routine. Consistency beats intensity when it comes to long-term success.

Now, let's talk about those days when time feels like a luxury you don't have. It's all about seizing opportunities. You got five minutes while you wait for dinner to cook? Do a quick set of squats. Are you watching TV? Use the commercial breaks for a living room workout session. These little bits of effort count and add up to more active time without you having to carve out large chunks of your day.

It's also essential to track your progress. Write down how long you've exercised each day or use a fitness app. seeing your workouts adds up over the weeks can be a powerful motivator. And remember to celebrate the small wins. If you've exercised a minute longer than yesterday, that's a win. It means you're moving forward, and that's what counts.

As you get comfortable with longer workouts, your goals evolve. You could start aiming for a 30-minute workout or decide to train for a 5K. Let your increasing stamina guide your ambitions. Fitness is a personal journey, and it should always align with what you want for yourself, not what someone else says you should do.

Ultimately, increasing your workout duration is about making exercise a non-negotiable part of your life, just like eating or sleeping. It's about finding joy in movement and challenging yourself to stretch your limits, bit by bit. So take it one minute at a time, and remember, every extra push is a step toward a stronger, healthier you.

The psychological benefits of regular, achievable workouts

Imagine getting into a routine where exercise isn't a chore but a regular part of your day that you look forward to. That's the sweet spot where the magic happens, not just for your body but for your mind, too.

Regular, achievable workouts can transform your mental state. Each drop of sweat is washing away a bit of stress. You feel more precise and sharper, almost like you've hit a reset button on your brain. It's that runner's high or that post-yoga bliss — it's natural and unique.

Exercise is like a natural antidepressant. It pumps up endorphins, those feel-good hormones that can lift your mood and keep it there. You don't need to be sprinting marathons to feel it, either. Even short, daily activities can boost your mood. It's about consistency, not extremes. When you've had a tough day, and you manage to squeeze in that workout, you've achieved something great and given your mind a chance to work through the stress, leaving you more relaxed and happier.

These small victories add up, especially on the rough days when dragging yourself off the couch feels impossible. On those days, just getting through your workout routine is a huge win, no matter how short. It proves you can overcome obstacles, building resilience beyond the gym. It quietly tells you, "If I can do this, what else can I tackle?" That kind of self-belief is gold.

Plus, there's the confidence boost. Every time you stick to your workout plan, you're keeping a promise to yourself. That's powerful. It builds trust in your ability to commit and follow through. As your strength and stamina improve, so does your self-esteem. You start seeing yourself as someone who can and does achieve goals.

And let's talk about the ripple effects. Exercise can improve your sleep, which is a game-changer for mental health. Better sleep means you're better at managing emotions, can think more clearly, and are more patient. It's like exercise sets off this positive chain reaction in your life.

It's not just about the endorphins or the confidence, though. Exercise is also about creating time for yourself. It's a break from work, family demands, and that never-ending to-do list. In those minutes when you're focused on your body and your breath, you're giving your mind a rest. It's meditation in motion.

There's also the social side of exercise. These connections matter, whether a nod of recognition from fellow early-morning joggers or a quick chat at a yoga class. They make us feel part of something bigger than our struggles. They remind us that we're not alone.

Regular, achievable workouts are a way of telling yourself that you matter. Your health matters. Your mental peace matters. It's not selfish to take that time; it's essential. And the beauty is that as your body grows stronger, so does your mind. That daily workout is more than just physical exercise; it's a vital part of your mental health toolkit.

So, when you think about the psychological benefits of exercise, it's not just about feeling good in the moment. It's about building a more robust, happier, more resilient you for the long haul.

Summary

- Regular exercise can significantly improve your mood and mental state.
- Achievable workouts, even if they're short, help reduce stress and anxiety.
- Consistent exercise releases endorphins, which are natural mood lifters.

- Sticking to a workout routine builds resilience and self-belief by proving you can overcome challenges.

- Regular physical activity boosts confidence through repeated achievement and improved physical fitness.

- Exercise can positively affect sleep quality, which benefits overall mental health.

- Exercise can serve as a form of meditation, providing a break from daily stress and helping to focus the mind.

- The social aspects of exercise, such as community and camaraderie, enhance emotional well-being.

- Committing to regular workouts is a form of self-care that emphasizes the importance of personal health and well-being.

- The discipline of exercise can create a foundation for building a more potent, more mentally stable, and happier life over time.

CHAPTER 10

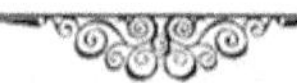

MANAGING MUSCLE FATIGUE AND RECOVERY

Take care of your body. It's the only place you have to live.

– Jim Rohn

Muscles screaming after those ten-minute bursts of energy? That's the sound of your body carving out a fitter, more robust you. But even superheroes need to rest. Chapter 11 dives into muscle fatigue and recovery, the unsung heroes of any workout plan. You grow by pushing your limits, but knowing when to ease off the gas is how you sustain that growth. Here, you'll learn not just to listen to your body but to hear what it's telling you about rest, repair, and readiness. Whether you're new to fitness or an old hand at the gym, this chapter will guide you through the best ways to manage muscle soreness, understand the signs of fatigue, and employ recovery techniques that set you up for your successive workout triumph. So, grab your water bottle, and let's get down to bouncing back.

The importance of rest and recovery in a workout regimen

You've been pushing hard, challenging yourself with every squat, press, and lunge. Your muscles are feeling it, and that's good – it means you're getting stronger. But what happens when you step off the mat? This is when the magic of rest and recovery comes into play, and it's just as crucial as the workout itself.

Think of it like this: when you work out, you put your muscles under stress, creating tiny tears in the muscle fibers. It sounds terrible, but this is precisely what you want because repairing these tears makes your muscles come back stronger. The repair process, however, can only happen when you need to work out. That's where rest days and recovery techniques steal the spotlight. They give your muscles the time to knit back together, stronger than before.

Rest days don't mean you're slacking off. They're an essential part of your workout routine, making your efforts count. Skipping rest can lead to overtraining, and that's a one-way ticket to exhaustion, decreased performance, and even injury. No one wants that. You might not see rest days as progress, but they are. They're the days when progress takes root.

Recovery isn't just about lounging on the couch, though that can be part of it. Active recovery is a gentle nudge to your muscles that keeps the blood flowing, helping to shuttle out waste products and nourish your muscles with oxygen and nutrients. Light walking, yoga, or a leisurely bike ride can do wonders and won't undo the hard work you've put in at the gym.

Sleep is another unsung hero of recovery. When you sleep, your body goes into overdrive, repairing muscles and replenishing energy stores. Cutting your sleep short is like leaving your car at the gas station with only half a tank when you have a long journey ahead. Not ideal.

Hydration and nutrition also play pivotal roles. Muscles need water and nutrients to heal. Think of food as your body's building material. If you want it to build a skyscraper, you better ensure you're giving it the good stuff. Protein is crucial here; it's like the bricks of your muscle building – without enough, recovery can't happen as efficiently.

Lastly, consider the power of stretching, foam rolling, or even getting a massage. They can increase flexibility, decrease soreness, and help your muscles be ready for whatever you throw at them next.

So, while it might be tempting to go hard every day, remember that rest and recovery are your partners in this fitness journey. They enable you to keep going, keep pushing, and get stronger. Listen to your body. Give it time to rest, and watch as it comes back more powerful for your next workout. That's the beauty of recovery - it's quiet but mighty.

Tips for recognizing and managing muscle fatigue

Muscle fatigue is like your body's own check engine light. It's a signal that something needs your attention. Ignoring it won't make it go away; it just means you could be setting yourself up for trouble. Learning to recognize and manage muscle fatigue is a skill that will serve you well, whether you're hitting the weights, pounding the pavement, or just living your daily life.

First up, know the signs. Your muscles might start feeling like they're made of lead; every lift and push is more of a struggle than the last. Or maybe they won't cooperate, shaking like a leaf in the wind when you try to hold a plank or press that dumbbell overhead. Pain is another red flag. We're not discussing the 'good burn' you feel when working out. This is different – it's sharper, and it doesn't quit when you stop the exercise. These are all your body's ways of saying, "Hey, can we take a breather?"

When you spot these signs, it's time to act. If you're in the middle of a workout, it might mean taking a more extended break between sets or calling it a day entirely. There's no shame in that. It's smart. Continuing to push through profound fatigue can lead to sloppy form, and that's when injuries sneak up on you.

Hydration is another crucial player in the fight against fatigue. Your muscles are like sponges; they don't work well when they're dry. But when they're hydrated, they're supple and robust. So keep that water bottle handy and sip regularly. It's a simple fix that can keep fatigue at bay.

Nutrition must be noticed, too. Your muscles need fuel to work, and they need the right kind of fuel. Carbs give you quick energy, while proteins are for repair and recovery. If you're skimping on either, fatigue will take hold faster. And remember about micronutrients like potassium, magnesium, and calcium. They're like the nuts and bolts holding the operation together.

Sleep is another non-negotiable. It's when your body hits the reset button. Shortchange yourself on shut-eye, and you'll feel it in your muscles. Aim for 7-9 hours a night to give your body the time it needs to repair.

And let's remember stress. It's not just a mind thing; it's a body thing, too. High pressure can make your muscles tense up and tire out more quickly. Find ways to dial down the stress – meditation, reading, a walk in the park. It all helps.

Lastly, don't skip those rest days. They're your body's chance to catch up on repairs. If you're feeling worn out, a rest day or an active recovery day with light movement can do wonders.

Remember, working out is just one part of the equation. Rest and recovery are just as important. Pay attention to what your body tells you; treat it right with good food, plenty of water, enough sleep, and the occasional break, and you'll be ready to tackle your next workout with gusto. It's all about balance. Keep your muscles happy, and they'll keep you strong and fit for all the activities you love.

Strategies for active recovery on rest days

Rest days are crucial, no doubt about it. But resting doesn't always mean you have to sit still all day. Active recovery is the secret sauce that can keep you moving and grooving without overdoing it.

Imagine this: You've been crushing it at the gym or on the track, and your body tells you it's time to ease up. That's when active recovery comes into play. It's about gentle movements that help your body heal without straining it further.

Think of activities that get your blood flowing but don't make your heart race. We're talking a leisurely walk through your neighborhood or a calm bike ride where you're not trying to set a personal best. Even a light swim can do the trick. The water supports your body and takes the pressure off while you move.

Yoga is another top pick for active recovery. It's like a triple threat—it helps with flexibility, core strength, and mindfulness all in one go. And you don't have to be a human pretzel to get the benefits. Just focus on stretching and breathing, and let your muscles thank you.

Stretching, in general, is a great way to spend your rest days. But don't bounce or push too hard. It's not about reaching your toes at any cost. It's about feeling a gentle pull and holding it, letting your muscles release any tension they've been holding onto.

And then there's foam rolling, which might be uncomfortable but can work wonders. It's like giving your muscles a massage. Slowly moving over various parts of your body can help break up knots and improve blood flow. Just remember, it's not a pain contest. If it hurts too much, ease off.

Remember fun activities like dancing or playing catch in the park. They can be part of active recovery, too. You're moving, you're laughing, and you're not thinking about reps or sets. It's a win all around.

Nutrition and hydration are still part of the equation on rest days. Drink water, munch on fruits and veggies, and ensure you're getting some protein to help with muscle repair. It's like refueling your car—good quality fuel makes for a smoother ride.

Listen to your body during active recovery. If something hurts, take it as a sign to slow down or try something else. It's a day to treat your body with kindness, not to push through discomfort.

In the end, active recovery is about balance. You are finding that sweet spot where you're helping your body heal without sliding back into full-on workout mode. It's a day to look forward to, not because you're going to crush calories, but because you're taking care of yourself so you can come back stronger for your next big workout. It's like a pause that refreshes, a chance to regroup and reset. And when it's done right, your body will feel rested, your mind will feel clear, and you'll be ready to tackle whatever comes next.

Summary

- Active recovery is essential; it involves engaging in low-intensity activities that promote blood flow and muscle healing without causing further strain.

- Gentle movements like walking, cycling, or swimming at a relaxed pace can significantly aid recovery.

- Yoga and stretching are beneficial on rest days for maintaining flexibility and reducing muscle tightness.

- Foam rolling can be a self-massage technique to alleviate muscle knots and enhance circulation.

- Enjoyable recreational activities, such as dancing or playing a casual sport, can also be part of active recovery.

- Proper nutrition and hydration should be maintained even on rest days to support muscle repair and overall recovery.

- Listening to your body is critical; discomfort or pain should be a signal to slow down or stop a particular recovery activity.

- Active recovery balances the workout regimen by providing necessary rest to the body while keeping it lightly active, setting the stage for a more effective return to training.

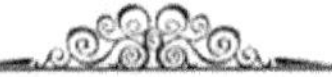

CHAPTER 11

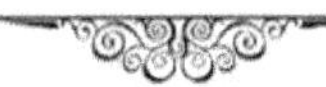

THE BENEFITS OF CONSISTENCY

Consistency might not sound like the most exciting word in the fitness dictionary, but it's the secret ingredient that can turn occasional, hard-earned sweat into tangible results. This chapter is about more than just convincing you that showing up matters. It's about understanding how the habit of regular workouts can transform your fitness journey and overall life quality.

Imagine your fitness goal is a giant rock. Each workout is a strike of the hammer. One hit won't make a dent, but a steady rhythm of strikes can split that rock in two. The power lies not in how hard you hit but in how persistently you strike. Similarly, working out consistently isn't about going all out in one session; it's the regularity that eventually sculpts the body and builds strength.

Let's break it down. When you exercise regularly, your body adapts. Muscles grow stronger, your heart gets more efficient, and your mind becomes sharper. It's like laying bricks for a fortress. Each session stacks up, making your body more resilient against illness and stress. While the benefits of a single workout are like a mood-boosting, endorphin-releasing magic spell, the regular casting of this spell builds a lasting enchantment of wellness.

You still have to grind every day. Consistency isn't about perfection. It's about setting a routine you can stick to. It could be a 10-minute morning routine, or it could be three yoga classes per week. What matters is that it's sustainable. It's about making exercise a fixed appointment in your calendar, something as regular as brushing your teeth.

When you keep at it, workouts become more efficient. Your body learns the movements, perfecting form and function, leading to better performance and less risk of injury. Your mind also gets in on the action; a regular workout schedule builds mental fortitude, chipping away at stress and anxiety. Over time, you'll find that missing a workout feels as odd as skipping a meal. It becomes part of who you are.

But it's not just about the physical and mental gains. Consistency in your workouts can ripple out into other areas of life. The discipline and dedication can cross over to work habits, relationships, and personal projects. It's like training wheels for your willpower, giving you the balance and strength needed to tackle life's ups and downs.

Remember, the benefits of consistency go beyond just getting fit or losing weight. It's about creating a balance that supports every part of your life. It's about setting a pace you can maintain long-term, not just for a sprint but for a marathon. And when life throws obstacles on your track, this consistent training gives you the agility and resilience to leap over them.

This chapter is a rallying cry for the power of showing up. It's a testament to the compound interest of fitness, where the steady investment of regular workouts pays off in a wealth of health benefits. It's not about being the best in the room; it's about being the best for you, over and over again.

The long-term health benefits of regular exercise

When you think about regular exercise, you might picture muscles and sweat. But it's so much more than that. Keeping up with a consistent workout routine is like a gift to your body that keeps giving, not just now but for years.

It starts with your heart, arguably the most important muscle in your body. Just like any other muscle, your heart gets stronger when you exercise. A strong heart pumps blood more efficiently, meaning every nook and cranny of your body gets the oxygen and nutrients it needs without your heart working too hard. This reduces the strain on your heart and can keep it healthy long into your later years.

But the benefits of a regular workout regime don't stop with your heart. Your bones get in on the action, too. Weight-bearing exercises, like running or lifting weights, tell your bones to bulk up, making them denser and reducing your risk of osteoporosis. That means fewer fractures when you're older and more confidence in your daily activities.

Your brain also loves it when you work out. Exercise increases blood flow to your brain, which can help spark the growth of new brain cells. It also releases chemicals that make you feel good and help keep your mind sharp. So, while taking care of your body, you're also caring for your mind, helping to ward off memory problems and keeping your thinking clear.

Then, regular exercise can help you maintain a healthy weight. It might seem obvious, but it's worth repeating: when you exercise, you burn calories, and when you burn more calories than you take in, you lose weight. But regular exercise means your body gets better at burning calories even when you're not working out, which makes it easier to keep the weight off.

But what does "regular" exercise look like? It doesn't have to be running marathons or lifting heavy weights. It can be as simple as a brisk walk, a bike ride, or a dance class — anything that gets your heart rate up counts. The key is to find something you enjoy so you'll keep doing it.

Regular exercise can also help you manage stress. When life's worries pile up, breaking a sweat can help bring them down to size. It's like hitting a reset button on your mood. Plus, finishing a workout can give you a sense of accomplishment, boosting your confidence and helping you feel ready to tackle whatever comes next.

Lastly, let's remember to sleep. Exercise can help you fall asleep faster and deepen your sleep. Getting enough good quality sleep is crucial for healing and repair, keeping your immune system in top shape, and even helping with weight management.

In essence, regular exercise is not just about being fit for the sake of it. It's about building a body that will take care of you for the long haul, a body that's more resistant to diseases, a mind that stays clear and focused, and a more vibrant life. So, while the immediate afterglow of a workout is great, the valid reward comes from the health and happiness that bloom over time, thanks to your dedication to staying active.

How consistency in workouts can lead to improved physical and mental health

Sticking to a workout routine is like planting a garden. At first, it takes a lot of effort to get things going, but with consistent care, you start to see the fruits of your labor over time. This is precisely how regular exercise works for your body and mind. You might overlook the benefits immediately, but with time and dedication, they grow and become a part of your life, enhancing it in ways you might not have imagined.

Imagine your body as a complex machine. Like any machine, its parts must move regularly to maintain good working order. Your body begins to operate more smoothly when you get into the rhythm of consistent workouts. Your muscles, including your heart, get more robust and more efficient. Climbing stairs or running for the bus isn't as tough as it used to be because your endurance is better. And with stronger muscles and better stamina, daily chores become more accessible, and you're less likely to get injured doing mundane tasks.

Consistency in workouts does wonders for your physical health, but the boost to your mental health is just as powerful. Exercise is a natural mood lifter. It releases chemicals in your brain that make you feel good, helping to reduce feelings of anxiety and depression. When you work out regularly, these chemicals give you a steady stream of feel-good vibes that can help you maintain a more positive outlook.

Think about the days you're stressed. Exercise can be a release valve for that tension. A consistent workout routine allows you to sweat out the day's frustrations, leading to a calmer, more centered you. This can translate to better sleep, too. When your head hits the pillow, your body is more ready to rest, and a good night's sleep is critical to both physical and mental health.

On top of all this, regular exercise has a ripple effect on other areas of your life. When you feel the benefits of your workout routine, you might be inspired to make healthier choices in other areas, like eating nutritious foods or cutting back on unhealthy habits. It's a cycle of good health that keeps on spinning.

Another big win for your mental health is sticking to a workout schedule. Every time you finish a workout, you've met a goal. This builds self-confidence and can motivate you to take on new challenges inside and outside the gym.

The most compelling benefit of consistent exercise is the long game. Diseases like high blood pressure, type 2 diabetes, and even some forms of cancer are less likely to show up in physically active people. By taking care of your body through regular workouts, you're not just living for today but investing in a healthier tomorrow.

Ultimately, the key to reaping these benefits is making exercise a regular, non-negotiable part of your life. It doesn't have to be hours at the gym or running marathons — it just has to be consistent. A brisk walk, a short bike ride, or even a dance session in your living room — if it gets your heart rate up regularly, it counts. As you build this habit, the rewards of your consistency are a healthier, happier you.

How small daily efforts accumulate over time

It might not seem like much when you start making small changes or taking tiny steps toward a goal. These little efforts won't amount to anything significant. But the truth is, they add up significantly over time. It's like saving money; one coin might not buy you much, but keep adding those coins to a jar, and one day, you'll find you've saved a small fortune.

In the world of fitness and health, the same principle applies. For instance, choosing stairs over the elevator every day might not make you break a sweat, but over weeks and months, it strengthens your leg muscles, improves your cardiovascular health, and can even help you shed a few pounds. Scientists and fitness experts back this up. Studies have shown that those who incorporate more walking into their daily life tend to have a lower risk of heart disease and better weight management.

Nutrition is another area where small daily choices add up. Swap out that sugary soda for a glass of water each day, and your body will thank you. You might not notice the change right away, but your body is receiving better hydration, and you're cutting down on empty calories. Over time, this leads to better skin, more energy, and potential weight loss. Research has confirmed that simply drinking water before meals can consume fewer calories and be a helpful tool for weight management.

The benefits of these tiny daily efforts extend beyond the physical. The brain also gets a boost from daily habits. For example, learning a new word every day might not make you a linguist overnight, but over months and years, it significantly broadens your vocabulary. Neurological studies show that learning new things can strengthen the connections in your brain, which is essential for long-term cognitive health.

This principle of small efforts leading to significant results is also seen in personal finance. If you save just a little from your paycheck every month, it might not give you the thrill of spending on something you want right now. But over the years, this habit can help you build a nest egg that might one day finance a home, a dream vacation, or a comfortable retirement. Financial advisors have long touted the benefits of regular, modest saving as a cornerstone of personal wealth-building.

Even relationships benefit from small, consistent acts. Sending a friend a message to check in, complimenting a loved one, or spending quality time on any given day can seem insignificant. But over time, these small gestures build trust, deepen connections, and strengthen our bonds with others. Psychologists affirm that the little things done consistently keep relationships healthy and fulfilling.

Every tiny action is a brick in the foundation of whatever you're building: fitness, knowledge, financial security, or relationships. The impact of these actions might take time, but they create a compound effect. As these small actions accumulate, they generate momentum, leading to surprising and profound changes over time. So, even when the progress seems invisible, remember that each small step moves you closer to your larger goals.

Summary

- Small daily efforts accumulate significantly over time, like saving coins in a jar, which leads to a large sum.

- Regular physical activity, such as choosing stairs over elevators, can improve leg strength and cardiovascular health with long-term benefits.

- Consistent healthy choices, like replacing sugary drinks with water, contribute to better hydration, energy levels, and weight management.

- Daily habits such as learning a new word daily can enhance your vocabulary and cognitive health.

- Even if small, regular savings can grow into substantial financial security, supporting significant purchases or retirement plans.

- Small, consistent acts in relationships, like checking in with friends or giving compliments, strengthen bonds and contribute to long-term relational health.

- The compound effect of daily actions generates momentum, leading to profound changes and progress toward personal goals.

CHAPTER 12

NUTRITION AND THE 10 - MINUTE WORKOUT

When pushing your body with short, high-octane workouts, eating right isn't just good advice—it's your secret weapon. Imagine your body's like a car. You wouldn't put just any old fuel in a racecar, would you? The same goes for your body. You'll want to fuel up smart to get the most out of those quick, intense sessions.

Before your workout, think quickly and lightly. A small snack that's got a nice mix of carbs and protein can give you a kick start without weighing you down. A banana with peanut butter or a small yogurt is like a pre-game high-five for your muscles.

Hydration is your best friend. Start sipping water a couple of hours before you plan to work out. Staying ahead of thirst is critical—you don't want to be playing catch-up when you're halfway through crushing your routine.

Right after the workout, your muscles are like sponges. This is your golden window. Within 30 minutes, try to get some quality protein and a bit of carb into your system. This could be a protein shake with a scoop of oats or a chicken sandwich. This isn't just refueling; it's getting ahead on recovery so you can return stronger.

Throughout the day, take advantage of veggies and fruits. They're not just vitamin treasure chests; they have fiber and enzymes that help your body handle the high-energy demands you're placing on it.

Fats are essential, but we're talking about the good guys. Avocado, nuts, seeds, and the oils from these foods are like long-burning logs on your metabolic fire. They help sustain your energy levels and keep you feeling full, so you're not tempted to dive into a bag of chips.

And speaking of temptation, processed sugar is a sly villain in the world of nutrition. Sure, it offers a quick energy spike, but it crashes just as fast, leaving you in a worse spot than before. It is better to rely on complex carbs like whole grains—they break down slowly, giving you sustained energy to keep the fire burning all day.

Let's remember to have regular meals. Consistent, balanced eating is your rhythm section—it keeps the beat for your body's energy levels. If you're skipping meals or eating erratically, your workouts (and mood) will feel it.

Lastly, rest days aren't cheat days. Thinking you can slack off on nutrition without sweating it out is tempting. But your body's still working, repairing, and prepping for the next challenge. So, even on rest days, keep your eating habits consistent with your goals.

All this isn't just fueling your workouts; it's investing in your health bank account. Good nutrition is a choice you make every day, and it pays off with interest in the form of energy, recovery, and overall well-being. And you don't have to be perfect. Even small, positive changes stack up over time, just like those high-intensity workouts you're crushing.

The role of hydration, protein intake, and quick energy sources

You've heard it a thousand times: "Drink water." But when you're all about squeezing every drop of benefit from your workouts, water is like the unsung hero of your fitness saga. It's not just about keeping a dry mouth at bay or avoiding that sluggish feeling. Proper hydration can differentiate between a good workout and a great one. Think of your body as a complex machine—water is the oil that keeps everything running smoothly. When you're well-hydrated, your heart pumps blood more efficiently, which means oxygen and nutrients get delivered to your muscles without a hitch.

Now, let's chat about protein. If your muscles could talk, they'd be constantly asking for it. Protein is what your body breaks down into amino acids, which then repair and rebuilds muscle fibers after you've been lifting, pushing, or pulling. Without enough protein, your muscles would be like workers without tools—unable to do their job correctly. After a workout, having protein is like giving your muscles a high-five and the tools they need to come back stronger.

But wait, there's more to the story. When you're in the thick of an intense workout, your body looks for quick energy to keep going. This is where carbohydrates come in. They break down fast into glucose, which your body uses for immediate energy. It's like throwing kindling on a fire for a quick flare-up of flames. A snack with simple carbs before exercise can be the ticket to power through those last few reps or that final sprint. But don't forget about complex carbs—like the slow-burning logs that keep the fire going, providing a steady energy source for the long haul.

But be careful with sugars. Sure, they give you a quick hit of energy, but it's like borrowing cash at high interest—you'll crash just as quickly, and your body will have to pay back the deficit. That's why it's wise to stick with natural, unprocessed sources for those quick-energy carbs like fruits. They come with their own natural fibers and nutrients that help balance out the sugar rush.

Your hydration game should still be firm when you're not working out. Your body constantly loses water through sweat, breath, and all the daily functions that keep you alive. So keep a water bottle handy and take sips throughout the day, not just when thirsty. By the time you feel thirsty, you're already playing catch-up.

Lastly, remember that hydration, protein, and carbs are part of the big picture. They work together like a well-oiled machine, helping you feel energized, perform better, and recover faster. It's about finding the right balance for your body and fitness goals. So, next time you prep for a workout or plan your meals, think about how water, protein, and carbs can work for you. It's not just about getting fit—it's about building a healthier, stronger you from the inside out.

Examples of quick, healthy meals and snacks

Fueling your body doesn't have to be a complicated science experiment or involve a fancy meal that takes ages to prepare. Sometimes, the best foods are the ones that are easy to make and don't require a ton of ingredients or time. These meals and snacks can keep you going, especially when life's busy, and you've got to fit workout and meal prep into your packed schedule.

You wake up groggy and need something to kick start your day. How about some Greek yogurt with a handful of berries and a sprinkle of granola? Greek yogurt is packed with protein, which is excellent for those muscles, and the berries give you that sweet kick plus some antioxidants without overloading on sugar. The granola? That's your texture and some extra fuel to get going.

For lunch, think about a turkey and avocado wrap. Grab a whole-grain tortilla, lay down some slices of turkey, and add some avocado for healthy fats and fiber. Roll it up, and you're good to go. If you want, throw some spinach or lettuce for some crunch and an extra serving of greens.

When it comes to dinner, stir-fries are a lifesaver. They're like the quick-change artists of the food world. You can throw in whatever you have in the fridge, add some chicken or tofu, and sauté with olive oil and soy sauce. Serve it over a bed of brown rice or quinoa, and you'll be full of nutrients and flavor without slaving away for hours in the kitchen.

Now, snacks are where many people get tripped up, but they don't have to be a diet downfall. Have you ever tried apple slices with a smear of almond butter? It's a game-changer. You get the natural sweetness of the apple with the creamy, nutty flavor of the almond butter, plus a nice dose of protein and healthy fats.

Another great snack is hummus with carrot sticks or cucumber slices. Hummus is made from chickpeas, which are high in protein, and the veggies are crunchy and hydrating. A snack feels like a mini-meal, keeping you satisfied until your next big plate.

If you're on the go, a small bag of mixed nuts can be a lifesaver. They don't require re; they're on, packed with protein, and healthy; they're super filling. Just be mindful of portion sizes because while nuts are good for you, they're also pretty dense in calories.

For those times when you're craving something sweet, dark chocolate can be your best friend. A few squares can satisfy that sweet tooth without sending your sugar levels through the roof. Plus, it's got a bit of caffeine, which can give you a slight energy boost.

All these meals and snacks are about keeping it simple, tasty, and nutritious. They prove that eating well doesn't have to be a complex many mountain of dishes to wash afterward. It's all about fresh, whole ingredients that give your body what it needs to stay energized and recover well, especially when balancing fitness with all the other stuff you've got going on in life.

Summary

- Combine Greek yogurt with berries and granola for a protein-rich start to the day.

- Use a whole-grain tortilla filled with turkey and avocado for a protein and healthy fats lunch.

- Create a quick stir-fry with various vegetables and a protein source like chicken or tofu, served over brown rice or quinoa for a nutrient-dense evening meal.

- For a snack, pair apple slices with almond butter for a satisfying crunch with a protein and healthy fat boost.

- Dip carrot sticks or cucumber slices in hummus for a fiber-rich, protein-packed snack.

- Carry a small bag of mixed nuts for an on-the-go snack full of protein and healthy fats, but be aware of portion sizes due to high-calorie content.

- A few squares can satisfy a sweet craving and provide a slight energy boost, thanks to its caffeine content.

- Focus on meals and snacks made from fresh, whole ingredients to maintain energy and aid in recovery.

- Emphasize the ease of preparation and the nutritional value of each food choice to fit into a busy lifestyle while supporting fitness goals.

- Remember the importance of drinking enough water, especially in high-intensity workouts.

CHAPTER 13

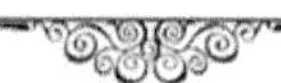

YOUR NEXT STEPS

The best time to start was yesterday. The next best time is now.

Embarking on a 10-minute workout journey is like unlocking a new level in a game where the rewards are genuine and all for you. It's about flipping the script on what exercise looks like and discovering that you can make a change that counts even in the small pockets of your day. Think of your day, the rhythm of your routine, and then picture this: just ten minutes carved out for you. That's less than the time you'd spend scrolling through your phone or waiting for your morning coffee to brew. Those ten minutes are a promise to yourself that you're worth the investment. Now, you might wonder if ten minutes can make a difference. But it's not about the time; it's about the action. Committing to moving your body with purpose for ten minutes daily ignites a spark that can light up your whole health picture. It's like the first domino that knocks down a chain of healthier choices. Starting can be as simple as choosing one exercise and setting a timer. You could jog in place, dance to your favorite song, or try a series of push-ups. Whatever you pick, it's about doing it with intention. Make those ten minutes count by focusing on your movements, breathing, and feeling alive in your body. And you don't have to go at it alone. Rope in a friend or family member, challenge each other and share the journey. Making it a shared experience can multiply the fun and the motivation. Before you know it, those ten minutes become a part of your connection with each other, too.

As days pass, you'll start to notice new strengths. You can do more push-ups than before, or you're out of breath less easily. Celebrate these wins, no matter how small; because every one of them is a step forward on your journey to a healthier you. What's great is that there's no deadline. There's no race to the finish line. This journey is yours, at your pace. And each day you choose to take those ten minutes for yourself, you're building a habit that can last a lifetime.

Sometimes, the hardest part is starting, but remembers, there's no such thing as perfect timing. Life is always happening, and waiting for the ideal moment might mean waiting forever. Your health and your well-being deserve to be a priority starting now. Those ten minutes? They're your daily act of self-care, your statement that says, "I am important." So, grab those shoes and find that spot in your living room, garden, or garage. Turn on the tunes that get you moving, and start. Ten minutes from now, you'll be glad you did. And who knows? In a week, a month, a year, you'll look back at this moment as the one that set you on the path to where you want to be. Not just physically but in the confidence and strength that comes from knowing you can and did do this for yourself.

Tips for maintaining motivation and measuring progress

Staying motivated and tracking your progress in your fitness journey is crucial, especially when you're committed to short 10-minute workouts. Here are some strategies to help you maintain motivation and effectively measure your progress.

First and foremost, set clear and achievable fitness goals. Having specific objectives, whether it's improving endurance, losing a certain amount of weight, or mastering a particular exercise, gives you something concrete to work towards. These goals serve as a source of motivation as you can visualize your success.

Consistency is critical to success in any fitness routine. Create a regular workout schedule that fits into your daily routine. Whether in the morning before work, during your lunch break, or in the evening, having a set time for your 10-minute workout can make it easier to stick to your plan.

Tracking your progress is essential. Consider using a fitness journal or a workout app to record the details of each workout. Note your exercises, the number of repetitions or duration, and how you felt during and after the training. This simple practice lets you see how far you've come and can be incredibly motivating.

Celebrate small victories along the way. Remember to acknowledge the power of owning your achievements. If you achieved a new personal best, completed a challenging workout without feeling overly tired, or made any progress toward your goals, celebrate it. Treat yourself with a healthy reward, or take a moment to reflect on your accomplishments.

Accountability can be a strong motivator. Partnering up with a friend, family member, or workout buddy who shares similar fitness goals can be a great way to stay on track. You can challenge each other, provide support on tough days, and celebrate your achievements together.

Variety is another tool to combat boredom and maintain motivation. Incorporate different exercises into your 10-minute routines. Try new things, whether a new yoga poses, another bodyweight exercise, or a fun dance routine. Mixing it up can make your workouts more enjoyable and engaging.

Visualizing your success can also boost motivation. Spend a few minutes each day visualizing yourself reaching your fitness goals. Visualization can make your goals feel more attainable, whether it's achieving your ideal weight, running that 5k race, or performing a perfect set of push-ups.

Setting up a reward system for reaching your fitness milestones can provide positive reinforcement for your efforts. Rewards could be treating you to a new workout outfit, a massage, or a weekend getaway. These incentives can make your fitness journey even more exciting.

Engaging with a fitness community in person or online can provide valuable support, encouragement, and a sense of belonging. Sharing your progress and challenges with others on a similar journey can help you stay motivated.

Beyond tracking your workouts, measure your physical progress as well. Take measurements of your waist, hips, and other target areas, and take photos at regular intervals. Sometimes, it's easier to see changes in pictures than on the scale.

Remember that progress takes time. Be patient with yourself, and keep going even if you don't see immediate results. Trust the process, and understand that consistency is critical to achieving your fitness goals.

Life can be unpredictable, and there may be days when you miss a workout or face setbacks. In such situations, it's essential to stay flexible and adapt. One missed workout only defines your entire fitness journey.

As you achieve your initial fitness goals, consider setting new ones to motivate yourself. Continuously challenging yourself with new goals ensures you always have something to strive for.

Periodically, take time to reflect on your fitness journey. Are you still excited about your goals? Do you need to adjust your workout routines or plans based on your progress? Self-assessment can help you stay on track and stay motivated.

In the world of fitness, motivation can be a fleeting thing. It's essential to keep your long-term goals in mind and utilize these strategies to maintain your enthusiasm for those short but impactful 10-minute workouts. Remember, small, consistent efforts over time significantly improve your health and fitness. So, stay motivated, stay consistent, and keep moving towards your goals.

How to advance to new fitness challenges over time?

Assessing your current fitness level is the first step. Understand where you are in terms of strength, endurance, and flexibility. This baseline helps you set achievable fitness goals tailored to your abilities and interests.

Setting clear and specific goals is crucial. Whether running a certain distance, mastering a yoga pose, or lifting a particular weight, having well-defined objectives gives your fitness journey direction and motivation.

Gradually increasing workout intensity is critical to progress. Add more weight, improve cardio intensity, or include challenging bodyweight exercises. This gradual approach prevents injuries and ensures sustainable improvement.

Variety keeps workouts exciting and prevents plateaus. Try different exercise types, such as interval training or circuit workouts. Changing things engages other muscle groups and challenges your body in new ways.

Learning new exercises broadens your fitness horizons. Explore different movements and techniques to keep your workouts fresh and compelling. Proper form and technique are essential, so consider working with a fitness trainer if needed.

Incorporating periodization into your routine involves breaking your training into phases, each with specific goals and intensities. This strategic approach optimizes gains and prevents overtraining.

Cardiovascular fitness is vital. Gradually increase cardio intensity and duration—transition from walking to jogging or incorporate high-intensity interval training (HIIT) to enhance cardiovascular endurance.

Functional training mimics real-life movements and improves daily functionality. Exercises like kettlebell swings and medicine ball throws enhance overall strength and stability.

Cross-training involves participating in various sports and activities. It prevents overuse injuries and adds variety to your workouts. For example, if you're a runner, try swimming or cycling.

Advanced training techniques like supersets, drop sets, and pyramid sets challenge your muscles uniquely, promoting growth and strength gains.

Recovery is crucial. Prioritize sleep, manage stress, and practice active recovery using foam rolling and light stretching techniques.

Professional guidance from a certified personal trainer or fitness coach can provide personalized plans and introduce advanced training methods safely.

Participating in fitness events or competitions related to your goals can motivate and offer a sense of accomplishment.

Stay patient and persistent. Fitness progress takes time and dedication, and setbacks are normal. Keep your eyes on your goals, stay consistent, and embrace the journey.

In our fast-paced world, finding time for fitness can often seem like a challenging task. The demands of work, family, and other responsibilities can make it feel impossible to prioritize our health. However, throughout the pages of this book, we've explored a powerful solution to this common problem—the 10-minute workout.

We began our journey by acknowledging the time-crunched lives that many of us lead. The daily hustle and bustle can leave us feeling overwhelmed and exhausted, leaving little room for exercise. But in those very moments when we feel like we have no time for fitness, the 10-minute workout shines as a beacon of hope. It's a manageable, realistic solution that fits even the busiest schedules. As we delved deeper, we uncovered the philosophy behind short workouts. We learned that science supports the effectiveness of brief, high-intensity sessions. Time efficiency became a central theme, highlighting that you don't need hours at the gym to achieve meaningful results. Short, focused workouts can be just as effective if not more so, than longer, less intense ones.

Setting realistic fitness goals was the next crucial step. We explored the importance of defining clear objectives aligned with our busy schedules. The SMART criteria became our guiding principles: specific, measurable, achievable, relevant, and time-bound. With SMART goals in place, we had a roadmap to follow, ensuring our fitness endeavors were both attainable and rewarding.

Creating personalized 10-minute workout plans became a practical skill we developed. From morning routines to quick office breaks, we discovered countless opportunities to integrate exercise into our daily lives. The versatility of these workouts allowed us to adapt them to our unique schedules and preferences.

We dove into the heart of the matter—the 10-minute workouts. We explored five distinct routines, each targeting different muscle groups, ensuring a balanced approach to fitness. We emphasized that these workouts were accessible to all, requiring minimal equipment—dumbbells and a weight bench. The exercises were simple yet effective, providing full-body training quickly.

However, the benefits of these short workouts extended beyond the physical. We explored how consistency in this routine can lead to a snowball effect. Starting with 10-minute workouts can build the habit and momentum needed to transition into longer sessions. The importance of managing muscle fatigue and recovery was discussed, emphasizing the need to listen to our bodies and avoid overexertion.

We also recognized that busy and working adults face unique challenges when it comes to fitness. Balancing work, family, and personal time can be demanding, but our 10-minute workouts provided a practical solution.

We offered insights into how nutrition complements this workout regime, stressing the importance of a balanced diet for optimal results. Success stories from genuine individuals who integrated 10-minute workouts into their lives were shared, showcasing the transformative power of this approach. These stories highlighted the positive changes experienced by people from various walks of life, reinforcing that anyone can reap the rewards of short, effective workouts.

In our penultimate chapter, we guided the next steps. We encouraged readers to apply what they've learned to their lives. We offered tips on maintaining motivation, tracking progress, and setting new fitness milestones. We emphasized that this journey is not about perfection but progress and consistency. And now, as we conclude this book, it's essential to reflect on the overarching message—that fitness is attainable for everyone, regardless of their busy lives. The 10-minute workout is not a quick fix or a shortcut to overnight success. It's a sustainable, practical approach to health and well-being that can fit into the rhythm of our daily lives. The benefits of consistency in our 10-minute workout routine cannot be overstated. We've learned that committing to these short workouts, even when life gets hectic, can profoundly change our physical and mental health. This consistency can become a cornerstone of our overall well-being, helping us navigate the challenges of our busy lives with resilience and vitality.

But it's not just about the physical gains. The psychological benefits of regular, achievable workouts are equally significant. Exercise can reduce stress, boost mood, and increase our overall sense of well-being. It can improve our self-esteem and provide a sense of accomplishment that carries over into other areas of our lives.

Throughout this journey, we've seen how small daily efforts can accumulate over time, leading to remarkable progress. These 10-minute workouts may seem modest, but their impact adds up exponentially. The key is staying consistent, motivated, and trusting the process. As the saying goes, "Rome wasn't built in a day." Similarly, our fitness and health are built over time, one A 10-minute workout at a time. In closing, this book has been a guide to unlocking the potential of 10-minute workouts. It has shown us that with determination, commitment, and a little creativity, we can make fitness a part of our daily lives, no matter how busy. It reminds us that our health is a precious gift that we must prioritize and nurture.

So, as we bid farewell to these pages, let us carry forward the knowledge and inspiration gained here. Let us embark on our 10-minute workout journeys, believing that small efforts can lead to significant change. Let us embrace the power of consistency, for it is the cornerstone of lasting health and vitality. In these final words of "10-Minute Fitness: Transform Your Day with Quick Workouts" by Paul Cannon, let's reflect on the journey we've taken together through the pages of this book. It's been a journey of discovery, empowerment, and transformation.

Throughout these chapters, we've explored the power of short, focused workouts to improve our lives. We've learned that fitness is not reserved for the few with abundant time but is accessible to all, regardless of our busy schedules. The 10-minute workout has emerged as a practical, realistic, and effective solution to finding time for exercise.

We've delved into the philosophy of short activities, understanding that science supports their effectiveness. We've set realistic fitness goals and learned how to create personalized 10-minute workout plans that fit seamlessly into our daily routines. We've embraced the importance of consistency, recognizing that small, consistent efforts lead to significant, long-term results. In our exploration of 10-minute workouts targeting different muscle groups, we've discovered that these routines are not only accessible but also adaptable to our unique needs and preferences. We've acknowledged the significance of managing muscle fatigue and allowing our bodies to recover. We've recognized that nutrition is vital in complementing our workout efforts. A balanced diet fuels our bodies for optimal performance and recovery. Real-life success stories have demonstrated the transformative power of integrating 10-minute workouts into our lives, showcasing the tangible benefits of improved fitness and overall well-being. In our penultimate chapter, we discussed the next steps—how to maintain motivation, measure progress, and set new fitness milestones. We emphasized that this journey is not about perfection but continuous improvement, consistency, and self-care. And now, in these final words, we stand at the crossroads of possibility. We hold within us the knowledge, the tools, and the inspiration to embark on our 10-minute workout journeys. We can prioritize our health and well-being and make daily choices that enhance our lives physically and mentally.

As we close this book, let us carry forward the belief that fitness is achievable, no matter how busy our lives may be. Remember that every 10-minute workout is a step toward a healthier, stronger, and more resilient version of us. Let us honor the commitment we've made to our well-being and the well-being of those we love. In these final words, let us find the motivation to take action, to lace up our sneakers, and to embrace the 10-minute workout as a powerful tool for positive change. Let us recognize that our health is a precious gift that we must nurture and cherish. As you enter the world beyond these pages, I encourage you to make fitness a lifelong companion. Let the lessons learned here be your guide, and let the 10-minute workout become a part of your daily routine. Remember, it's not about the time you spend but the dedication you invest in yourself. In conclusion, fitness is a journey of self-discovery, resilience, and transformation. It's a journey that continues beyond the confines of this book. So, my friends go forth with confidence, determination, and the knowledge that you can transform your day with quick workouts.